D0942037

The Krisiloff Anti-inflammatory Diet

*The Prevention for
Urinary Problems,
Heartburn, Arthritis, &
Potentially Prostate Cancer.*

Milton Krisiloff, M.D.

ONE WORLD PRESS
Prescott, Arizona

ISBN: 978-0-9777356-3-1

Cover Design, Text and Layout Design:
Adi Zuccarello, www.adizuccarello.com

This book was printed in the USA by:
ONE WORLD PRESS
1042 Willow Creek Road
Prescott, AZ 86301
800-250-8171
production@oneworldpress.com
www.oneworldpress.com

PREFACE

The advice, information and directions presented in this book are not intended to replace professional medical care and evaluation. In medicine, many serious problems can initially present as minor complaints. Readers should consult a doctor on all matters relating to their health and well-being. It is important that a thorough medical evaluation be obtained before starting on the Krisiloff Diet. No action or inaction should be taken based solely on the contents of this book. Readers who fail to consult with appropriate health care professionals assume the risk of any injuries.

The author assumes no liability or responsibility for any loss, real or perceived, or any damage caused or perceived to be caused, directly or indirectly by the information in this book.

DEDICATION

I dedicate this book to my wife, Flora and my children Kevin, Scott and Matthew, for all the love and understanding that they have given me. From them, I have mastered the strength of listening and compassion that make being a doctor so special. I would also like to thank Flora for all the hours she has shared with me to make this book possible.

ABOUT DR. KRISILOFF

Dr. Milton Krisiloff grew up in New York City and earned his undergraduate degree at Trinity College in Hartford, Connecticut. In 1970, he earned his medical degree at the Chicago Medical School in Chicago, Illinois.

In 1971, he completed his medical internship at L.A. County - U.S.C. Medical Center in Los Angeles, California. For the following two years, he was a medical officer with the United States Navy serving both aboard ship in Vietnam and at the Naval Medical Center in Oakland, California.

From 1973-1977, he did his residency in urology at Columbia Presbyterian Medical Center in New York City. Columbia Presbyterian Medical Center is considered by many to be amongst the top five urology training centers in the United States.

Since 1977, Dr. Krisiloff has practiced urology in Santa Monica, California. Throughout these years, he has been closely involved with Saint John's Hospital in Santa Monica. Saint John's is known to be one of the preeminent medical centers in the United States.

For many years, Dr. Krisiloff served as the Chief of Urology at Saint John's Hospital. In 1988, he was elected as the Secretary of the Medical Staff at the hospital. He went on to be elected the Vice President of the Medical Staff, and then from 1990 to 1991, he was elected the Chief of the Medical Staff of Saint John's Hospital.

From 1988 to 2004, Dr. Krisiloff served as the personal urologist to Ronald Reagan, 40th President of the United States ---an honor that Dr. Krisiloff considers to be the highlight of his medical career.

In 1991, Dr. Krisiloff was highlighted in Los Angeles Magazine as one of the top ten urologists in Los Angeles. He has served in the practice of urology for 30 years.

TABLE OF CONTENTS

1: INTRODUCTION

This book is intended to share my great success with the Krisiloff Diet ---an all natural, anti-inflammatory diet. The diet has been successful for almost 30 years in helping thousands of my patients find cures for their common chronic medical problems. With a purely holistic approach, I have helped patients cure problems associated with the urinary tract, digestive tract and rheumatoid arthritis. Cardiac problems, sinus conditions, chronic headaches and even some with elevated blood pressure have been helped as well. Additionally and importantly, it might even be a way to prevent the most common cancer in men --- prostate cancer.

Until now, there has been little help and little hope for many people suffering from these common everyday medical problems. The quality of their life is compromised, and they are frustrated because they cannot find solutions. Despite billions of dollars spent by our health care systems, millions still suffer.

This book is for people who cannot find answers and hopefully show them that many of their medical conditions can be avoided or cured by living with a healthy diet. It will also show that many unnecessary tests, unnecessary medications and unnecessary surgeries can be avoided. It is not intended to replace consultation with your physician. I always recommend that when symptoms first develop, you should consult your doctor to ensure that serious medical problems do not exist.

I have practiced medicine as an urologist for 30 years. Early in my career, I began searching for more effective ways to help cure certain common urinary problems, because I and many other urologists knew the usual standard treatments were not working. Even today, urologists often express frustration in treating certain common urinary problems because of their lack of success in helping these patients. They often confess it would be fine with them if they never had to see these groups of patients. Yet the opposite is true for me. With my diet, I know I can cure these patients.

People often ask how I discovered this successful program for so many different conditions. My answer comes from the ancient medical instruction: "Doctor, listen to your patients." Through listening carefully to my patient's observations, I came to understand the underlying cause of their problems, and I was able to formulate an approach that could cure them.

When I first started in urology, there was a painful, largely unsuccessful method to treat women with a chronic urinary problem called urethral stenosis or urethral syndrome. It involved dilation, or stretching, of the tube that carries urine from the bladder. The procedure was very painful and usually achieved only short-term relief. As a young doctor, I wanted desperately to find a better solution for these women.

Fortunately for me and for the thousands of my patients who followed, a patient informed me that she noticed a definite correlation between her urinary symptoms and certain items in her diet. Then several other patients added to my knowledge with their observed relationship between their problems and their dietary intake. From this information, I was able to formulate the Krisiloff Diet to first cure urethral syndrome and then so many other urinary problems.

Over time, I observed the diet having great success in men with prostatitis --- a condition which affects close to 45 million men. Then I found success in treating women with urinary incontinence. It also worked to cure children who were wetting their bed. In the last 10-15 years, I have used the diet in areas of prostate cancer detection and prostate cancer control.

Use of the Krisiloff Diet grew as my patients reported many secondary gains. Patients noticed that their urinary problems were being cured along with many of their other chronic medical problems. Heartburn, irritable bowel and rheumatoid arthritis were being cured as well.

Patients with heartburn or acid reflux no longer needed medication. Patients with chronic headaches, even migraines, had significant improvement or even complete resolution of their headaches. Patients with rheumatoid arthritis, especially in the early stages, were seeing their pains disappear. Chronic sinus conditions and certain types of heart palpitations went away. Adult onset asthma, often caused by acid reflux, was being cured. People with "restless leg" syndrome no longer had this problem.

As medical science learns more about the role of inflammation in causing disease, I realize I have discovered a simple, highly effective method to help many different problems --- a success which comes from essentially a natural anti-inflammatory diet. I have come to understand that difficult and complicated ways are often not the best answer. With the Krisiloff Diet, I believe I have found the "Holy Grail" explanation for inflammation, and the ways to prevent its devastating impacts.

With this knowledge, I hope to rescue millions of people from their pain and frustration with many common medical problems, and at the same time, help to save billions of dollars in unnecessary health care costs.

I also hope to explain how the Krisiloff Diet might help prevent prostate cancer, the number one cancer in men today. Prostate cancer is estimated to affect 1 in 6 of all men, a cancer that kills 29,000 men annually.

2: INFLAMMATION

Today as the concept emerges that chronic inflammation causes many common medical problems. I believe I can demonstrate empirically that the Krisiloff Diet can help prevent or cure these problems because of its special anti-inflammatory properties. My belief is that the Krisiloff Diet is the "Holy Grail" explanation for preventing inflammatory diseases, and that chronic inflammatory condition can be prevented or cured with dietary changes only. For the last thirty years, and through experiences with thousands of my patients, I have seen dramatic cures. Through this book, I hope to show you how this is possible.

In normal circumstances, the inflammatory response is used by our bodies for protection. With inflammation, blood cells called macrophages surround the area of injury. It is the job of the macrophages and their chemicals to help the body repair damaged tissues. We need the acute inflammatory reaction to stop the disease process. Problems develop however if a chronic inflammatory response occurs. A response defined as one that goes on for many months or even years --- not just for a few days.

The inflammatory response produces substances called oxygen free radicals. In the acute situation, these molecules help destroy cells attacking the body. However when the inflammatory reaction becomes chronic, the oxygen free radicals become less effective. Rather than destroying cells, they only damage the cells. A damaged cell has a higher potential for mutation, and therefore is more likely to cause problems such as chronic disease or cancer.

Inflammation has been linked to stomach, liver and colon cancer. There is now a belief that inflammation can also be linked to prostate cancer. Studies also suggest that cancer patients have improved survival when inflammatory reactions can be controlled. Cancer growth slows in an anti-inflammatory environment. Recently, a large study was underway to see if the anti-inflammatory drug Vioxx could help cancer patients. Unfortunately, these studies had to be stopped because people using Vioxx to treat their arthritic conditions, had increased incidences of heart problems and strokes.

Chronic inflammation has also been implicated in heart disease and heart attacks. C-reactive protein is a non-specific blood test marker for inflammation because C-reactive protein blood levels increase in response to inflammation. Cardiologists believe that increased levels of C-reactive protein can predict individuals with higher risk for heart disease. Recently, people have suggested that even Diabetes and Alzheimer's disease can be linked to inflammation.

To help my patients better understand the importance of the Krisiloff Diet and its association with inflammation, I use the analogy that certain foods and drink cause an "allergic" inflammatory response. It is important to realize that if they go on the diet, problems disappear ---if they go off the diet, medical problems return. There seems to be a direct link between the Krisiloff Diet and the cause and the prevention of inflammatory diseases.

3: HOW THE KRISILOFF DIET WORKS

The Krisiloff Diet ---a simple, holistic cure for many different medical problems, essentially functions as an anti-inflammatory diet and has been used clinically with great success for almost 30 years in thousands of my patients.

In the 1990s, to quantify my observations, I examined almost 2,400 charts of patients from my medical practice. The medical records of 1710 men with prostatitis and 675 women with urethral syndrome (all treated with dietary restrictions only) were reviewed. No medication or surgical manipulation was used. For patients on the Krisiloff Diet, 87% of men and 89% of women were cured of their urinary problems. These results proved for me that their problems stemmed from what I call an "allergic-like inflammation" caused by caffeine, alcohol, and hot spicy foods, and it showed that the Krisiloff Diet was highly effective.

The patients ranged in age from 18 to 83 years old and all had at least two or more symptoms associated with either their prostatitis or urethral syndrome. The symptoms included discomfort with urination, frequency of urination or the need to urinate multiple times during the night. Other symptoms were urgency to void, a loss of urine called urgency incontinence, or continuation of urine dribbling after the person thought they should be finished. Testicular pain, lower abdominal pain, groin pain and perineal pain were also some of the symptoms.

Two associated symptoms existed in 25% of patients. Three or more symptoms were found in 75% of patients. Patients were treated with a dietary approach that demanded total abstinence from caffeine, alcohol, and hot spicy foods. Then all patients were reevaluated for their symptoms at the end of 12 weeks. They were carefully instructed to avoid these "forbidden items" and to maintain 100% compliance as even a slight deviation could prevent resolution of their symptoms. Success was based on the patient's self-evaluation of their symptoms at the end of 12 weeks. I considered my approach successful if each of their individual symptoms had disappeared.

The achievements of the Krisiloff Diet came from curing the irritation caused by specific foods and drinks. Its success came from my realization of the major role irritants play in causing many medical problems.

Patients must be educated regarding caffeine, alcohol, and hot spicy foods. Many think caffeine is synonymous only with coffee. But caffeine is also found in tea, decaffeinated coffee, decaffeinated tea, cola drinks, some non-cola drinks, and in chocolate. Caffeine-free herbal tea or grain beverages are acceptable drinks.

Eliminating alcohol means all alcohol, including beer and wine. Forbidden hot spicy foods include salsa, red pepper, hot mustard, horseradish, chiles, Tabasco sauce, pepperoni, curry and wasabi.

It is not necessary to be on a bland diet. Mild spices such as salt, black pepper, onion, salad dressing or ketchup are not irritants and are acceptable. Some people have been told by physicians to avoid tomatoes and citrus juice. I have not found this necessary, and tell my patients it is okay to consume these products.

I stress to my patients that caffeine, alcohol and extremely hot spicy foods cause the symptoms by an "allergic-like" reaction leading to inflammation. For the great majority, avoidance of these irritants leads to complete resolution of their problem. To "cheat" on the diet or not follow it completely 100% of the time might only prolong symptoms or cause the symptoms to flare again.

People often ask if they have to stay on the diet permanently. If they want to never have symptoms again, the answer is yes. Their problems are specifically caused by an "allergic-like" reaction to caffeine, alcohol and hot spices. If they choose not to be on the diet they have a good chance of experiencing symptoms again. Some people can be so sensitive that they go months or years without symptoms, but then, if they go off the diet for even 1-2 days, they will have an immediate recurrence. Others can go back to the "irritants" in moderation and may not have immediate problems, but can have their problems recur over time.

I am often asked which one of caffeine, alcohol or hot spices is worse than the others. I have seen people try all permutations. Unfortunately, all three are equal in their ability to cause the problem. Eliminating two categories and staying on one does not seem to help most people.

The relationship of food allergy and disease has been considered by physicians in the past. This is the first time however that a specific program, The Krisiloff Diet, is being proposed to help cure so many different medical conditions, and perhaps be a key component in the prevention of prostate cancer as well.

Why do people choose to stay on the Krisiloff Diet permanently? Firstly, it is because it has eliminated serious, chronic conditions that have plagued them. Secondly, the great majority of people tell me the quality of their life improves dramatically. Most people notice that after only a few weeks on the diet, they feel better than they have felt for years.

In summary, the Krisiloff Diet eliminates inflammatory reactions in many different systems of the body. By using the diet, it is my hope that millions of patients will benefit, and billions of dollars in health care costs will be saved. These specific dietary irritants (caffeine, alcohol and hot spicy foods) appear to represent the long-sought explanation for many of the most common problems in medicine today.

4: WHAT BRINGS PEOPLE TO THE UROLOGIST

Every year millions of people suffer from problems related to their urinary tract system, yet these problems are rarely discussed. Most of these people believe that their urinary problems are unusual and unique to them. In reality, they suffer from some of the most common problems in all of medicine. Among these problems are prostatitis, urethral syndrome, urine incontinence, epididymitis, bed-wetting, premature ejaculation and a fear of prostate cancer.

A 1977 study by the U.S. National Center for Health Statistics revealed that 25% of the visits by men to urologists are for prostatitis and that approximately 50% of all men experience symptoms of prostatitis during their lifetime. Similarly, 50% of women have an attack of urinary symptoms at some time in their lives.

The symptoms which bring both men and women to the urologist can be very similar. The clinical symptoms may be of an irritative nature, a painful nature, an obstructive nature or may present as blood in the urine. If you have any of these types of urinary symptoms, I urge you to consult your physician to make sure a serious problem is not present. Fortunately, most of the time, there isn't one. To better understand the various symptoms let me give you a brief description and example of each category.

Irritative symptoms are most commonly represented as increased urinary frequency, burning with urination, urgency to void or urgency incontinence. During the day, an average person will urinate approximately once every 3-4 hours. If someone suffers from urinary frequency, he or she may go to the bathroom to void every 60 to 90 minutes, sometimes even every 30 minutes.

When there is discomfort or burning with active urination, dysuria is the medical term used to denote these symptoms. The patient frequently complains of an unusual awareness of discomfort during the passage of urine. Unfortunately, the normal act of voiding becomes a major ordeal.

If a person has urine urgency, the signal to void will usually come on very suddenly and the ability to control the need to urinate can be completely lost. In a normal situation, we receive a signal to urinate and then we can hold the urge until the appropriate time. If someone suffers from urgency, he or she just can't wait. The individual has to race to the bathroom immediately and will often wet their pants. This is described as urgency incontinence. An additional irritative symptom can be a post-void dribble or urine drops in the pants after the person thinks he or she is finished urinating.

Painful clinical symptoms present as pain in different locations of the body. Some people complain of pain in the lower abdomen, the lower back or the inner thighs. For women, pain on sexual intercourse or pain in the vaginal area can be associated with urological problems. For men, pain after orgasm or pain in the testicles can be the complaint.

Obstructive symptoms to the urinary stream form the third category of clinical problems which causes people to seek out a urologist. These symptoms include hesitancy, which is defined as the delay associated with initiating the act of urination. People may have to wait 15-20 seconds before the urine will come. Some complain of a feeling of incomplete emptying of the bladder, which means that they urinate and a few minutes later they feel that they have to go again. Others are bothered by a urinary stream which is interrupted or flows in spurts, and may even spray. Nocturia (getting up more than once a night) for either men or women is considered abnormal and is another sign of not emptying the bladder completely.

Blood in the urine is called hematuria. This is the fourth general category of symptoms which cause individuals to see their doctors. There are two classifications of hematuria. The first is microscopic hematuria, meaning blood is only seen by the doctor under the microscope on urine analysis. Fortunately, this is the most common type of hematuria and in the majority of cases it is not associated with any significant problem. The second form is called gross hematuria, which is when blood is seen in the urine without the aid of a microscope. The patient is the one who sees the blood in the urine in the toilet bowl. Although gross hematuria may represent insignificant problems, in many cases it is associated with serious medical problems. Therefore, people who see gross hematuria must be thoroughly evaluated by their urologist.

Hematuria Case Experiences

Ellen is a 64 years old employment agency owner. She complains of having to urinate all the time. In the daytime, she urinates every one to two hours. At night she gets up from her sleep three to four times to urinate, and she also complains of pain in the lower abdomen.

Ellen became frightened when she started to notice some blood on the toilet paper she used to wipe herself after urinating. Because of the bleeding, she agreed to have a cystoscopy exam to evaluate her bladder.

The cystoscopy showed some inflammation of the urethra but the rest of the bladder was perfectly normal. From this exam, I was able to diagnose a urethral syndrome. I immediately placed her on the Krisiloff Diet.

One month later, she came back to see me and all her symptoms were gone. She no longer had to get up at night. The pain in the lower abdomen was gone. She was now only urinating in the daytime every three to four hours, and there was no longer any blood on the tissue.

Alan is 43 years old and runs his own investment company. He has a long history of blood in the urine which can only be seen with a microscope (microscopic hematuria). He also urinates frequently and gets up four times a night to urinate.

He is very disturbed with his urinary problem because it is interfering with his work and his life. The frequent daytime urination makes it difficult to sit through meetings, and he is extremely tired because he cannot get a good night's sleep.

Because of the blood in the urine, he had been evaluated by two previous urologists with an x-ray of the kidneys and a cystoscopy. Both urologists agreed that he had prostatitis, but no treatment was working for him.

When Alan saw me, I placed him on the Krisiloff Diet. Five weeks later, his frequent daytime urination was gone. He now gets up only once each night and a urinalysis shows he no longer has any blood in his urine.

5: THE MALE AND FEMALE URINARY SYSTEMS

I am presenting a brief, simple description of the urinary tract in both men and women to help make the understanding of the problem easier.

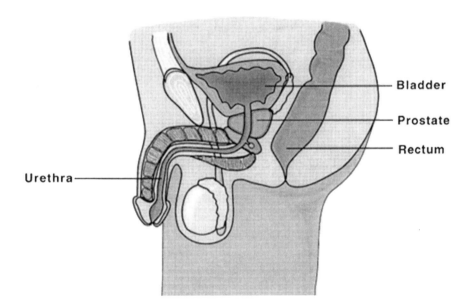

A Schematic Illustration of the Male System

Urine is produced by the kidneys and travels down the ureter tubes to the bladder. The bladder stores the urine and later evacuates it, first through a channel in the prostate gland and then through the urethra. The function of the prostate gland is to produce fluid and enzymes for ejaculation. The prostate rests against the rectum, so a urologist can easily feel the prostate during a digital rectal exam. All men should be evaluated and examined by a physician whenever they have urinary problems.

During this digital rectal examination, the prostate should feel soft. If it feels hard, an individual has to worry about the possibility of prostate cancer. Although the prostate gland normally enlarges with aging, the size of the prostate does not correlate with urinary symptoms. Some men with the largest prostates have no symptoms. Some men with very small prostates can occasionally stop urinating completely.

More often than most doctors realize, common urinary symptoms can be caused by an inflammation of the prostate which is not caused by an infection. More importantly, this inflammation can occur at any age. I have seen it start in children as early as 6-7 years of age and as late as people in their 70s and 80s. This condition is called prostatitis. The inflammation is caused by diet and produces the patient's troubling symptoms of frequency, urgency, burning and/or getting up many times at night. These symptoms can easily be reversed without the need for any surgery, medication or herbs.

In women, the urethra is located just above the vagina. The urethra is the channel for urine to pass out from the bladder. A woman's urethra is much shorter in length than a man's urethra. Because of the shorter distance to the bladder, a woman can develop infection more easily than a man because it is easier for bacteria to travel from the vagina to the bladder. However, in many instances urinary symptoms in women are not caused by infection. Instead, they are usually the result of inflammatory changes in the urethra. This common condition in women is called the urethral syndrome and the inflammation is caused primarily by dietary allergic reactions. This syndrome is common in all age groups, from the preteens to the 80s. Sometimes the symptoms are caused by vaginal douching or the use of bubble bath. Here again, the symptoms can be eliminated by diet alone without any need for medication or manipulation and, of course, eliminating douching or bubble baths.

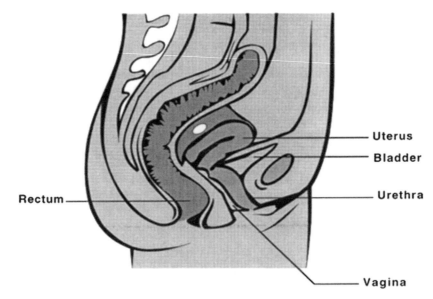

A Schematic Illustration of the Female System

6: PROSTATITIS

Prostatitis is essentially divided into two clinical categories: acute prostatitis and chronic prostatitis. Approximately 25% of annual visits by men to a urologist are for prostatitis. It is estimated that 50% of all men will experience symptoms of prostatitis during their lifetime. Clearly it is a major health problem and can severely impact the quality of men's lives.

With acute prostatitis the patient experiences a high fever, shaking chills and a sudden onset of urinary symptoms such as burning and frequency. A urine culture will show bacterial infection. Often the man feels he is suffering from "flu." The urologist finds a tender, swollen prostate on rectal exam. The patient feels very ill, but it is a relatively easy condition to treat. It can usually be cleared in just a few days with proper medication.

Chronic prostatitis represents greater than 95% of prostatitis conditions effecting men. It represents inflammation rather than infection and does not often respond to antibiotics. There is no evidence to suggest that prolonged courses of antibiotics are beneficial and many different attempts to link a specific bacterial organism with prostatitis have been unsuccessful. The problem can plague men for months or years, and it is always difficult to find a solution.

The clinical symptoms of chronic prostatitis for individuals vary but include frequent daytime urination, frequent nighttime urination, lower abdominal pain, pain in the inner thighs, pain in the urethra or referred pain to the tip of the penis. Pain after ejaculation, blood in the semen (hematospermia), urinary urgency, pain in the rectum, pain in the testicles, the inability to stop the urination at the end of the stream (post-void dribble) and hematuria (blood in the urine) either at the beginning or end of the urinary stream can also be seen.

In a study of over 1700 men in my medical practice, I found that men with chronic prostatitis complain of multiple symptoms. The most common symptoms were urine frequency (31%), nighttime voiding (25%), burning (14%), urgency (13%), testicular or penile pain (12%), microscopic hematuria (11%), hesitancy or interrupted stream (7%), pain with ejaculation (4%), post-void dribble (4%) and hematospermia (3%.)

Most Common Symptoms In Men With Prostatitis

- Urine Frequency *31%*
- Nighttime Voiding *25%*
- Burning *14%*
- Urgency *13%*
- Testicular / Epididymal Pain *12%*
- Microscopic Hematuria *11%*
- Hesitancy / Interrupted Stream *7%*
- Pain With Ejaculation *4%*
- Post-void Dribble *4%*
- Hematospermia *3%*

There is no evidence that antibiotics work, but traditionally, the treatment for chronic prostatitis is to place men on antibiotics anyhow. Another method is prostatic massage, where a rectal exam by the urologist milks the prostate vigorously. This can go on once a week for months. Unfortunately, it can become quite expensive and, again, there is no proof of its benefits.

The Krisiloff dietary approach in my study of these 1700 men has shown a cure rate of 87% for men with chronic prostatitis.

Although recently, there has been some acceptance of the Krisiloff Diet by my medical colleagues, I am fond of telling the story of when I first presented my findings at an international conference on prostatitis held at the National Institute of Health in 1999. There were urologists from around the world, and when I finished my presentation there was dead silence. The overall perception was that few, if any, of my colleagues believed what I had to say. That evening at the cocktail party many came up to me and jokingly holding out their alcohol or spicy hors d'oeuvres said "I guess this is not on the Krisiloff Diet."

I left the conference wondering why there should be such resistance to a simple approach which is highly successful, costs nothing and shows results in as few as 4-6 weeks. My message to them was simply to try my approach first and if it doesn't work, if there are no results in 8-12 weeks, then we can use all the traditional methods urologists have been trained to perform.

I concluded that the problem of their lack of acceptance appeared to be twofold. First, after years of intense training, very few medical professionals seem willing to accept something so simple. Secondly, there may be underlying monetary concerns. These patients return many times to their urologist without resolution of their problem --- often spending large amounts of money with little benefit. Many tests, procedures and even surgeries are performed and the economic remuneration to the doctors is significant -- especially if the pathway to cure is complicated and protracted.

I hypothesize that if the Krisiloff Diet was widely accepted, then perhaps half of the Urology practices in American would no longer be needed.

Prostatitis Case Experiences

Saul is a 57 year old businessman with a history of chronic prostatitis for several years. His problem involves urine frequency where he goes to the bathroom every 60 to 90 minutes in the daytime and three times at night. He wakes up from his sleep to go to the bathroom and because of this, he complains of being tired all of the time. He also suffers from post void dribbling. Whenever he thinks that he has finished urinating, he has to wait an additional 30 to 60 seconds to make sure that drops do not wet his underwear or stain his pants. His final symptom is not always present but is very bothersome when it occurs. He suffers from urine urgency which means that when he feels like he has to urinate, he has to stop everything he is doing and rush to the bathroom or he will wet his pants. The feeling of urine urgency comes on so suddenly and so forcefully at times, that he feels that he can not control the ability to hold back his urination.

Before seeing me, he had seen another urologist and had been tried on several medications to try and shrink the size of his prostate, and also to relax his bladder to try and get rid of his symptoms. Unfortunately, nothing worked, and he was told he would need to have prostate surgery.

Saul was referred by a friend to see me. After a thorough exam and laboratory tests, I confirmed that he had prostatitis. However, rather then recommend surgery, I put him on the Krisiloff Diet. Eight weeks later, all of his urine symptoms were gone. As you can imagine, he was extremely happy because all his chronic symptoms disappeared, and he no longer had to worry about having surgery.

Frank is a 43 year old physician who needs to urinate frequently. In the daytime he urinates every 1-1/2 to 2 hours, and also has a burning sensation with urination. On my digital rectal exam, I felt a firmness in the right side of the prostate. A urine test showed no infection, and his prostate specific antigen test (PSA) was normal.

I discussed with Frank that his symptoms most likely suggested a prostatitis. Prostatitis can make the gland feel firm and abnormal. I also explained that in some cases of prostate firmness, cancer could be a possibility. But before rushing to do a biopsy, I suggested he go on the Krisiloff Diet for one month, and then return to have the rectal exam repeated. If the Diet worked, the prostate inflammation and firmness would be gone, and there would be no need for a biopsy. If however after one month, the firmness was still there, he would need a biopsy to check for cancer.

He went on the Krisiloff Diet and one month later, all his urinary symptoms were gone. More importantly the prostate exam was completely normal. The firmness was gone.

Steve is a 48 year old mechanic who has a 20 year history of on and off bouts with prostatitis. His main problems are pain in his groin and pain after ejaculation. He confesses to me that he is not enjoying sex, because he is always worried about pain after ejaculation.

He has seen other urologists in the past and has been tried on multiple antibiotics. Once he even stayed on an antibiotic for three straight months. Still there was no relief.

When he came to see me, I found no infection in his urine. On my digital rectal exam, I felt a very swollen prostate. It was much larger than would be expected for someone his age. I started him on the Krisiloff Diet, and within 6 weeks, the pain in the groin was gone. Within 10 weeks, he had no more pain with ejaculation. Also the size of the prostate on rectal exam was now 50% smaller than what it had been 10 weeks previously. The reason for the shrinkage was that the chronic inflammation previously present had caused the prostate to swell, and now that the inflammation was gone, the tissue was no longer swollen or inflamed. The prostate had returned to its normal size.

Steve has stayed on the Krisiloff Diet, and in the last four years, he has not had any recurrence of his symptoms. He tells me now that his "sex life is great!"

Letter from F.A.

Dear Dr. Krisiloff,

I hope you find the following helpful.

My initial bout of prostatitis occurred when I was in my mid-twenties. The symptoms: groin pain, difficulty in urination, etc. were painful and sometimes downright unbearable. The first urologist I consulted with, (a "top man" in my area), promptly put me on a rigorous antibiotic regimen that lasted several weeks. This yielded partial results, however, within a month or so the symptoms came back. After a battery of tests to determine that this was indeed a benign condition, I was again put on an antibiotic regimen. Over the next year and a half, I was kept on "antibiotic maintenance", i.e. I took the pills daily for months on end! All the while the symptoms were on-again, off-again. I took one antibiotic in particular for so long that I finally developed an allergic reaction to it. My urologist's answer, a different antibiotic! By this time, I was becoming very depressed. I was truly feeling plagued. It was about this time that I decided to make a change and rather than try a different antibiotic, I decided to see a different doctor.

Luckily for me, I was referred by my G.P. to Dr. Krisiloff. His credentials were impressive; Chief of Urology at St. Johns Hospital in Santa Monica, rated top in his field by Los Angeles Magazine in their issue on L.A.'s best doctors. Nonetheless, I remained skeptical but committed to finding a different approach that would yield true results and give me some long term relief. Dr. Krisiloff's approach was indeed different. During my initial consultation, he in effect confirmed what I already knew, that antibiotic therapy (the generally medically accepted treatment for prostatitis) is largely ineffective in treating this condition. Secondly, he outlined a program for me to follow, one that included among other things certain life-style changes. Again, I remained skeptical for a short while, since the results were not necessarily over-night. However, several months into the program, I was in fact symptom free, and more importantly, I remained symptom-free! So how do I know that it is Dr. Krisiloff's program that has helped me? Very simply, go off the program (and I did after a year or so of being symptoms free) and the symptoms return.

Dr. Krisiloff has been my urologist for over 10 years now. His program has enabled me to take charge of my own health and moreover my life once again. His approach is innovative and yet atypical of the usual medical model thinking......
Thank goodness!

Note*: In this and subsequent chapters, I have included letters from patients I have treated over many years. Because of the sensitive nature of some of the symptoms, the patients, identities remain anonymous, although, the patients gladly consented to the inclusion of the letters in this book.

7: URETHRAL SYNDROME

Urethral syndrome is an inflammation of a woman's urethra, and this annoying medical problem is the counterpart to men's prostatitis. It is a major health problem which is not well understood by most doctors and is often mistaken for bladder infection. This syndrome can severely interfere with the daily quality of a woman's life. Individuals with urethral syndrome will commonly complain of urinary difficulties. Additionally, because of the location of the urethra, many women complain of pain in the lower abdomen or vagina or pain on sexual encounter. A woman should be diagnosed with urethral syndrome when she has urinary symptoms and no infection can be found in her urine. The most common individual symptoms in women with urethral syndrome parallel that of men with prostatitis.

Before I discuss the urethral syndrome, I must further mention bladder infections because they, too, are common in women although possibly not as common as the urethral syndrome. Urethral syndrome is often mistaken for a bladder infection. However, there is one major difference between the two, although the symptoms can be exactly the same for both. A bladder infection, which is called acute cystitis, is a true infection demonstrated by a positive bacterial culture of the woman's urine. Bacteria must be present in acute cystitis on the urine culture. In urethral syndrome, which is an inflammation and not a bacterial infection, the urine culture does not show bacterial infection. Therefore, there is no reason for the use of antibiotics in the urethral syndrome. It is not an infection and, therefore, will not respond to antibiotics. It is an inflammation and another approach other than antibiotics must be used.

The most common cause of acute cystitis (a bacterial infection) is sexual intercourse when vaginal bacteria is pushed into the bladder via the urethra. To prevent cystitis after intercourse, it is very important that women get up in the 5-10 minutes following sex and urinate. Early urination will empty the bacteria that has been introduced into the bladder. However, if the woman fails to urinate in a timely manner, the few bacteria introduced into the bladder with sexual activity will multiply into many and lead to an infection.

Another important means of preventing cystitis is for women not to do vaginal douching or to clean the vaginal area mechanically. The process of douching again forces bacteria into the short urethra and causes a bacterial infection. Bubble bath should also be avoided. Simply cleaning the vaginal area in a daily shower or bath is adequate hygiene and will prevent the possibility of bacterial infection associated with douching.

Another important means of preventing bladder infection in women is wiping oneself properly after a bowel movement. A woman should never reach between her legs and wipe from back (from the rectum) to front. This will only bring rectal contamination towards the vagina and urethra and allow bacteria to accumulate where it eventually can be introduced into the bladder. Wiping after urination should always be from front to back away from the vagina. To wipe after a bowel movement, the hand should be placed behind the buttocks at the rectum and the wiping movement should be up and away toward the lower back so that the bacteria cannot be moved into the vaginal area.

One final word about cystitis: some women do everything as described above and still get bacterial infection. In this case, it is recommended that the women continue to use the preventive measures described above but, in addition, they should be placed on what doctors call a post coital (after sexual intercourse) low-dose antibiotic. After sex, the woman should get up to urinate and then take a very low-dose antibiotic pill. This prevents infection in many persistent cases of truly recurrent bacterial infections. Women who are unable to prevent cystitis with the previously mentioned natural methods should talk to the urologist about this low-dose antibiotic program, where a pill is taken after sexual activity only.

In a study of 675 women in my medical practice, I found that most women with urethral syndrome complained of more than one symptom when they came to see me. Frequent urination was the most common symptom (34%) followed by nocturia (23%), urgency (21%), dysuria (19%), urgency incontinence (10%), microscopic hematuria (10%), lower abdominal or vaginal pain (8%), and the feeling of incomplete emptying (8%.)

Most Common Urinary Symptoms For Women With Urethral Syndrome

- Urine Frequency *34%*
- Nighttime Voiding *23%*
- Urgency *21%*
- Burning *19%*
- Urgency Incontinence *10%*
- Microscopic Hematuria *10%*
- Lower Abdomen / Vaginal Discomfort *8%*
- Feeling of Incomplete Emptying *8%*

As previously mentioned, in urethral syndrome, there is never evidence obtained of an infectious process. Bacteria are never found on urine culture, which means that antibiotics are useless. Out of frustration and in search of a treatment for the syndrome, doctors have tried many different approaches but, unfortunately, nothing has worked.

A commonly used approach in the past is urethral dilation. In this procedure, the urethra is stretched with a progression of increasingly larger metal tubes. The results are usually painful for the patient and offer little to no relief and can be costly. It was in searching for an alternative to this approach that I was able to originally develop the Krisiloff Diet.

Chronic antibiotic administration has also never been shown conclusively to work. Studies have looked for unusual bacterial organisms to be linked to urethral syndrome but none have ever been definitely isolated. Biofeedback and psychological counseling have also been advocated but never proven to be significantly worthwhile.

Additionally, estrogen creams have been used by many women since it is also believed that an estrogen deficiency is responsible for these symptoms. However, here again no long-term results have ever been achieved.

In my practice, the Krisiloff dietary approach has cured 89% of women with urethral syndrome.

Urethral Syndrome Case Experiences

Wendy is a 34 year old housewife who has been complaining of a severe burning sensation in her urethra for the past year. When she came to see me, she was feeling very depressed. She had seen another urologist whose examination had found that her urethra was severely inflamed. Tests of her urine showed no signs of infection. Her former urologist had treated her for a possible yeast infection, but the treatment was of no help. He thought she might have a venereal disease, but all her tests for venereal diseases were normal. He told her she needed to lose weight, but that too was of no help.

When she came to see me, she was thoroughly frustrated. She confessed to me that her urinary problem was beginning to interfere with her daily routines. It was becoming more difficult to concentrate and to take care of her family.

I explained that many doctors do not understand the relationship between diet and severe inflammation in the urinary system. I suggested the Krisiloff Diet. She was hesitant at first that something so simple might work, but nothing else had worked, so she was willing to give it a try.

After being on the Krisiloff Diet for four weeks, she came back to see me. She felt about 60 - 70% better. I again encouraged her to stay on the diet and return in another four weeks. When she came back, after a total of eight weeks on the Krisiloff Diet, all her problems had disappeared. Her life was back to normal and she was forever grateful.

Melissa is a 34 year old woman who complains that she has to go to the bathroom all the time, and yet when she goes, very little comes out. She is constantly in the bathroom in the day and nighttime. She has a long history of burning with urination and recurring pains in her urethra.
When Melissa came to see me, she had already seen two previous urologists who had put her through a series of urethral dilations. The dilations were not helpful, and now she was being told that she would need a formal operation to open her urethra wider.

I explained to her that I do not believe in urethral dilations and that today most urologists are of the same opinion. I explained that it was this very procedure that led me to find an alternate way to treat people with chronic urinary problems.

My early experience with the urethral dilation, as a young physician, showed me that not only was it very painful to the woman, but that it also did not work to relieve symptoms in most patients for more than just a few weeks. I stopped performing this procedure for women when I first started using the Krisiloff Diet.

'   I placed her on the Krisiloff Diet and within one month she was cured of all her symptoms.

Letter from D.G.

My first visit to Dr. Krisiloff was about seven years ago to get a second opinion as to the necessity of surgery which was scheduled for by my urologist, who was treating me for a very sore and painful urethra and bladder. This Beverly Hills doctor told me "surgery is the only way to get better."

Dr. Krisiloff examined me and took a urinalysis. I was in disbelief when I was told that I did not have a bladder infection, nor that I needed any surgery. Dr. Krisiloff then explained to me that I have urethral syndrome, and to get better all I need to do is cut out caffeine, spicy foods, chocolate and alcohol from my diet. I had seen many urologists over the years and would always receive at least two prescriptions "to get better". Sometimes remaining on medications for months, and still not getting relief from my symptoms.

After following Dr. Krisiloff's advice and changing my diet, and giving up my coffee breaks, within a month, I was better! My symptoms do return when I start drinking my much loved coffee.

I am very grateful to Dr. Krisiloff for saving me from having a very unnecessary surgery, and finally putting to an end my many years of pain, discomfort and the constant urge to use the restroom.

Sincerely,
D.G.

Letter from D.A.

To Whom It May Concern:
Because of the very uncomfortable burning sensation in my urethra, I went to see my Doctor. He found blood in my urine and suggested I see a urologist. This is what brought me to Dr. Krisiloff. He examined me and also my urine, with the same findings.

He inquired about my eating and drinking habits. What impressed me about Dr. Krisiloff was that he did not prescribe any medication. Instead, he told me: no coffee, no chocolate, no alcohol and no spicy foods for three months. After this time, I should return to see him. I stuck to this diet faithfully and within two weeks the burning sensation had disappeared. I returned to Dr. Krisiloff after the three months period and the result was no more inflammation of the urethra and no more blood in my urine. Of course, I miss my coffee and chocolate but the bottom line, meaning my health is more important to me. What a great way to solve a problem!

Thank you, Dr. Krisiloff.
Sincerely,
D.A.

Letter from S.J.B.

Dear Dr. Krisiloff,

I had a whole host of urinary problems, including frequency during the day, nocturia as many as three times nightly, and sometimes I didn't quite make it to the bathroom at night. When I developed a burning sensation, I knew I was in trouble.

I was examined by a freshly-minted physician, obviously quite intelligent and very caring. She found microscopic hematuria (blood in the urine) and prescribed a one-week course of an antibiotic. Although urine culture revealed no infection, when I returned after the course of antibiotics she again found microscopic hematuria. Again, urine culture revealed no infection. Baffled, she referred me to Dr. Krisiloff, who promptly explained to me - and presumably her - about urethral syndrome, a condition which affects approximately 40 million American women.

I was stunned. How could this fresh, bright young physician not know about such a widespread problem? And the solution was equally stunning: no caffeine, no alcohol, no hot spicy foods (not a problem - spices have never been my friends), and no chocolate. No Coca-Cola? No chocolate? No, not so much as a taste.

In a way I was not surprised that these substances were the cause of the blood in my urine: my father, a dermatologist who practiced for 50 years, always said that coffee was the most allergenic substance on the planet.

8: URINE INCONTINENCE

It has been estimated that urine incontinence affects 13 million Americans and adds $16 billion a year to health care costs.

The urinary bladder stores urine and holds it until it is time to be properly released. By definition, urine incontinence means the involuntary loss of urine at inappropriate times, resulting in wetting of the patient's clothing. It is important to realize there are three main types of urine incontinence and that the causes and treatment for each are vastly different.

Stress incontinence is a situation almost solely in women, where the women lose urine in active situations such as laughing, coughing, sneezing, jumping or running. Men can suffer stress incontinence but this is usually in situations where they have undergone surgery for prostate cancer and are left with stress incontinence similar to women in this particular situation.

The pathophysiology behind stress incontinence in women can be two-fold. First, the anatomical position of both the bladder and urethra changes because of multiple pregnancies or because of a previous hysterectomy. The changes result in an abnormal pushing out, or protrusion, of the bladder and urethra. Secondly, the intrinsic ability of the urethra to close becomes defective. When these situations occur, the abdominal pressure on the bladder from coughing, jumping, running or laughing cannot be counteracted by the usual forces on the urethra which keep the tube closed and prevent leakage. The normal anatomical positions or functions have changed, therefore, urine leaks or spurts out.

This type of situation (stress incontinence) can only be corrected with surgery that elevates the bladder and urethra back into their normal position so that pressures are equalized and there is no leakage of urine. Fortunately, stress incontinence is not as common as women and doctors think and, therefore, surgery for incontinence can and should be avoided in most instances unless the stress incontinence is shown to be the dominant form of incontinence in the individual's clinical situation.

Urgency incontinence is a loss of urine when the feeling of the need to urinate comes on so quickly that one cannot get to the bathroom in time. Urgency incontinence can be pure and be the only form of incontinence, or it can be a mixed type of incontinence that is also present with the above-described stress incontinence. The patient must understand that stress incontinence can be fixed with surgery but urgency incontinence will have no improvement with a surgical procedure. In many cases, it may even get worse. Therefore, one must determine specifically if the main problem is primarily of a stress nature or is of an urgency type. Urgency incontinence is also associated with other urinary symptoms such as frequency and nocturia. These are symptoms which one does not experience with the type of stress incontinence that requires surgical correction.

If a woman has a component of urgency incontinence and knowing that this will not be corrected by surgery, it is very important that the woman not agree to surgery until the Krisiloff Diet has been tried. However, in many cases women are persuaded to have surgery. The unfortunate situation results in unnecessary surgery with no improvement in these symptoms. Surgery for urgency incontinence should be avoided at all costs.

In men urgency incontinence is associated with prostatitis but the occurrence of urgency incontinence is not nearly as common as in women. Urgency incontinence can also be associated with neurological disease and is especially common after a stroke. If this condition occurs after a stroke, medications can sometimes be effective for control.

Overflow incontinence is the final but least common type of incontinence. In men it is usually caused by an enlarged prostate gland which does not allow the bladder to empty. The bladder contains large amounts of urine that does not empty with voiding so that the urine spills like water over the top of a glass which continues to be filled. Individuals with incontinence must have a bladder volume check to be sure they do not have overflow incontinence.

Most instances of urgency incontinence are due to inflammatory changes in the man's prostate or the woman's urethra. These inflammatory changes are caused by the allergic-like reaction to dietary products and can easily be cured with the simple use of the Krisiloff Diet.

Urine Incontinence Case Experiences

Vivian is a 75 year old woman who works as a hospital volunteer. As soon as she feels the urge to urinate, she has to rush to the bathroom because the urge is too great. Her problem is urgency incontinence. Within seconds of getting the signal to urinate, she has to reach a toilet, or the urine will leak out. Unfortunately, in most instances, there isn't enough time to get to the toilet, so she wets herself. As you might imagine, she is greatly concerned by the smell of urine in her undergarments, and the constant need to wear protective pads. It truly interferes with her lifestyle.

After a careful evaluation, she was placed on the Krisiloff Diet. One month later, the wetting and the smell were gone. She could not believe how simple the cure was.

Miriam is a 46 year old housewife who leaks urine periodically throughout the day. The leaks occur often, and she is never aware of when it is going to happen. She has absolutely no warning --only panic, when she suddenly realizes that she has lost bladder control and is wet again. Her loss of urine is not brought on by coughing, sneezing or strenuous physical activity. She suffers from incontinence.

Her physical examination revealed a mild dropping of the bladder which was the result of several previous pregnancies. I explained to her that in this exact situation, many other urologists would recommend surgery. I told her that women with her symptoms and physical findings are never cured with surgery, because the operation would be done for the wrong reasons. I emphasized that she should avoid surgery, because her type of incontinence was not caused by the bladder dropping.

I placed her on the Krisiloff Diet, and six weeks later, she came back to see me. The leakage had completely stopped. She no longer was wetting herself, and she has been forever grateful.

Letter from V.S.

Dear Dr. Krisiloff:

Sorry I have to "write" this letter, but my computer died yesterday.

I wish to thank you for curing my incontinence without surgery; now I have dry panties and outer clothing. This was accomplished by your diet, i.e., no tea, coffee, soft drinks, wine, liquor or chocolate.

It's just wonderful! Thank you very, very much.
Sincerely and gratefully,
V.S.

Letter from A.F.H.

Dear Dr. Krisiloff,

It was rather fascinating to hear what you had to say last week. Since I saw you, last night was the first night I slept through until 9 a.m. without getting up to urinate.

I spent a whole lifetime (91 years!) like a camel, never got up at night, could go about 8-10 hours during the day with no problem. Then, from one day to the next, boom! All hell broke loose. I thought perhaps my bladder had fallen as there was no control at all. For the first time in my life, I wore pads. Neither coffee, alcohol nor spices had ever affected me. Why so suddenly? It didn't make sense. Now I must say that the results speak for themselves.

Sincerely,

A.F.H.

9: ENURESIS (BED-WETTING)

Enuresis is the clinical name for bed-wetting. Although enuresis can affect people of all ages, it is mostly a problem that occurs in children and adolescents. It is also more common for the problem to occur in boys.

It is estimated that 5-6 million children and adolescents suffer from bed-wetting. When a child wets the bed at age 6, or if he or she has stopped bed-wetting for a period of time and then resumes bed-wetting, it is considered a problem.

There are two types of enuresis. Primary enuresis means the problem occurs solely at night. Diurnal enuresis is defined as having urine symptoms such as frequency, urgency and urgency incontinence in the daytime and bed-wetting at night. Anyone with primary enuresis should have a physical exam and urine analysis to rule out a medical problem. A person with diurnal enuresis should have a more extensive evaluation to make sure there are no significant medical problems that may be presenting as bed-wetting. This evaluation usually involves ultrasound to evaluate and make sure there are no anatomical problems with the kidneys or bladder.

Traditional therapy for bed-wetting is with either a drug or non-drug approach. The drug approach uses oral medications or nasal sprays to stop the bed-wetting. Medications can be effective about 30-50% of the time but, like most medical therapy, they are expensive and do have side effects. The non-drug approach is either with behavioral therapy, such as hypnosis or an alarm system which wakes the child when they begin to wet themselves. These methods also are successful about 30-50% of the time but they too are expensive.

The Krisiloff Diet is just as successful as the above approaches to eliminate bed-wetting in all ages. It works in 40-50% of cases. Because it is simple and inexpensive it should always be considered the primary treatment option for enuresis and the more aggressive approaches should be considered only if the Krisiloff Diet is not successful.

Bed-Wetting Case Experiences

Sophia is a 9 year old girl who wets her bed. She has been on multiple medications with no help. She most recently was placed on a nasal spray called DDAVP which is a potent medication that functions as an anti-diuretic to retain fluids. It often is successful, but in this case there were no positive results.

Sophia saw me and was placed on the Krisiloff Diet. When she was seen one month later, she was not wetting the bed. Her mother said, "It was like a miracle."

Craig is a 7 year old boy who suffers from bed-wetting. Except for the bed-wetting, he has no other urinary symptoms. Both he and his parents are very concerned. He feels sad that he can't spend the night over at his cousin's house because he worries that he will wet the bed. He is embarrassed that it might happen.

They have tried a monitoring system to try to stop him from wetting the bed. The system consists of a pad and an alarm. The alarm goes off when the pad starts to get damp. Unfortunately, the method is not successful.

After examining Craig, I placed him on the Krisiloff Diet, and after one month, there was no change. I urged Craig and his parents not to give up. I explained that it might take up to twelve weeks to see results. If it did not work by twelve weeks, only then would I consider it an unsuccessful treatment.

Four weeks later, there was great improvement. Now he was only wetting the bed once or twice per week --- not every night. It became much easier for Craig and his parents to believe in the Krisiloff Diet. Indeed, one month later, the bed-wetting stopped completely, and it has never resumed.

Erik is 14 years old and has been a bed-wetter all his life. His father is convinced that it is psychological, and they both are very frustrated. The boy himself is very embarrassed, and you can only imagine how it has interfered with his life --- no sleep-overs, no camps. He has even reached the point where he will get up in the middle of the night and hide the wet sheets to keep from feeling ashamed.

Erik started the Krisiloff Diet, and within eight weeks, great things had happened. He stopped wetting the bed, and for the first time, he could enjoy spending the night with his friends.

10: EPIDIDYMITIS AND TESTICULAR PAIN

Epididymitis is a common ailment in men. The epididymis is a gland that sits alongside the testicle and is where sperm undergoes metabolic changes after it leaves the testicle.

In epididymitis there is an inflammation of the epididymis so that men complain of testicular pain with some pain moving into the groin area. There can be swelling alongside or within the testicle itself. The pain can be dull to very severe and can often be chronic in nature. The situation is not a threat to fertility but can be very debilitating and frightening because many men think it might represent testicular cancer.

Epididymitis can often develop because of underlying prostatitis. The prostate becomes inflamed and the inflammation travels through the tubular structures connecting the prostate and the epididymis and results in pain and possible swelling.

Here again diet plays a major role in causing the problem and with simple dietary adjustments the problems can disappear.

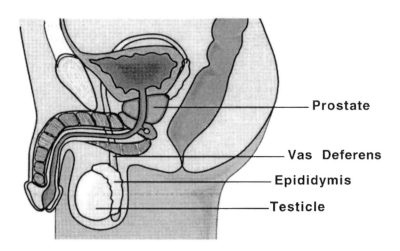

A Schematic Representation of the Male Reproductive System

Epididymitis Case Experiences

Joseph is a 40 years old actor who has had pain in the right testicle for several months. He also has pain with ejaculation.

When I examined him, I found the testicle itself was normal. But during the exam, he felt tenderness behind the testicle at the spot where the epididymal gland is located.

I put Joseph on the Krisiloff Diet, and five weeks later, all the tenderness was gone. His pain with ejaculation was gone too. He was not placed on antibiotics or anti-inflammatory medications as is often done by other urologists. He was treated with the Krisiloff Diet only, and five weeks later all his symptoms were gone.

Carl is a 32 years old businessman who had seen another urologist in the past for a six month history of prostatitis. But still his symptoms recur. He has come to see me because of difficulty with urination and pain in the testicle. I placed him on the Krisiloff Diet, and within six weeks, all his symptoms were gone.

Two years later, Carl came back to see me. He confessed that because he was feeling well, he went off the Krisiloff Diet "to see what he could get away with." This time when I examined him, I not only found severe pain behind the testicle but a swollen epididymis as well. He went back on the diet, and one month later, all the pain and swelling were gone.

11: PREMATURE EJACULATION

Premature ejaculation is defined as the inability of a man to hold his ejaculation long enough to satisfy his partner. In many, the man will ejaculate in as little as 30 – 45 seconds after arousal. Premature ejaculation is estimated to effect 20% to 40% of men --- about as common as those who suffer from erectile dysfunction. As one can imagine, studies show great stress and marital difficulties for couples with this problem. 50% of these couples are reported to have interpersonal problems resulting from their problematic sex lives.

In my experience, men who suffer from premature ejaculation frequently have an underlying problem with prostatitis. Seminal fluid is produced by the prostate as well as glands called seminal vesicles. A prostate irritated by inflammation allows ejaculation to occur quickly.

Today, there are medications to help control premature ejaculation. They are effective about 30% to 40% of the time. Unfortunately, they are expensive and have side effects including possible suicidal tendencies.

Rather than medication, I first use the Krisiloff Diet for premature ejaculation to treat the underlying possible chronic prostatitis. This natural approach is simple with no side effects. The diet's success rate for cure is 30% to 40% --- no different from the medication. You will know within a matter of weeks if the diet is succeeding or if a different approach needs to be tried.

Premature Ejaculation Case Experiences

Charles is a 50 year old businessman who has had a problem with premature ejaculation for three to four years. He is very concerned, and his wife is becoming very frustrated. His problem is starting to affect their marriage.

When I examined him, the prostate felt normal. He told me that his only urine symptom was that he would get up once every night to urinate. I placed him on the Krisiloff Diet and within eight weeks, the premature ejaculation disappeared. He and his wife remain forever grateful.

Richard is a 38 year old worker in the movie industry. He has had a history of premature ejaculation for several years. Richard is a single man, and his problem is creating quite a disturbance in his life.

In addition to the premature ejaculation, he feels that he is urinating too frequently, and at times, it is difficult to start his urine stream. He has to wait 20 to 30 seconds to start the urinating. He has seen other urologists in the past and has been treated with multiple antibiotics. Unfortunately nothing has worked.

Richard came to see me, and after a complete evaluation, I placed him on the Krisiloff Diet. One month later his urinary problems were gone, but he still had premature ejaculation. I told him not to despair, that it would take more time, and I encouraged him to stay strictly on the diet. Six weeks later, he came back to see me. He was excited to report that the premature ejaculation was now no longer a problem.

12: PSA SCREENING FOR PROSTATE CANCER AND THE KRISILOFF DIET

Since the late 1980s, the "PSA blood test" has entered the vocabulary for millions of men. Prostate-specific antigen (PSA) is a protein produced by the prostate gland, and is used as a blood test in screening patients for prostate cancer. While PSA blood levels are not specific indications of prostate cancer, they are considered a good screening test, because they have a relative high degree of sensitivity to indicate if prostate cancer exists.

Other conditions originating in the prostate (besides cancer) can elevate PSA blood levels. Benign prostate hypertrophy (BPH), an enlarged prostate associated with aging, can cause an increase in PSA. Chronic prostatitis, an inflammation of the prostate gland, can produce an elevation in the PSA level in many patients. A recent urinary tract infection even after treatment can also elevate the PSA for as long as four to six weeks.

Due to various causes of PSA elevations, scientists are constantly looking for a better test, with a higher degree of certainty, to specifically detect cancer. The hope presently is for a blood test called Early Prostate Cancer Antigen (E-PCA) which will be far more specific to detect prostate cancer. Early results are encouraging, but as of now, it is still not available as a routine clinical test.

People often ask if there is a problem to draw blood for a PSA test after a rectal exam or after sexual activity. They are concerned there could be an erroneous elevation in these situations. However, studies in these situations where the blood is drawn immediately prior, and immediately after, show that PSA value rises no more than 0.1 ng/ml in value; a rise of no clinical significance.

The normal accepted range for PSA blood levels is between 0 ng/ml to 4 ng/ml. Some urologists believe that the range should be lowered to 2.5 ng/ml for men in their forties and fifties. They believe that lower values will lead to earlier investigation and therefore cancers will be found at an earlier stage of development. Thus the chance for cure could possibly be better with earlier intervention. Those opposed to the lower values however are concerned that there would be a significant increase in the number of unnecessary biopsies due to this lowered range. Additionally, even if cancer was detected at this earlier stage, many of these patients might never need treatment because they could be in a group where their cancer could potentially stay dormant for the rest of their lives.

PSA blood tests are recommended starting at age 50. However, if the patient has a father or brother with prostate cancer, or if the patient is African American, then the PSA screening should start at age 40. There is an increased risk for families with a history of prostate cancer. Also, African American men have a higher risk for prostate cancer then Caucasian or Asian men.

Besides yearly blood tests, men should also have a yearly rectal exam. With this exam, the normal prostate feels soft and smooth. In prostatitis, the prostate can feel spongy or boggy. If the gland feels hard or irregular, one must consider the possibility of cancer. A prostate exam should always be done in conjunction with the PSA blood test because 20% of men with prostate cancer can have a normal PSA value.

Men often ask what a normal prostate or a cancerous prostate feels like. I use the analogy of pushing on the tip of one's nose and feeling the soft cartilage. This is what a normal prostate gland feels like. But pushing on the bony surface of the forehead reveals a firm to hard area, and this is what a cancerous prostate could feel like.

When the possibility of prostate cancer exists, an ultrasound and biopsy of the prostate are recommended. For this procedure, a probe is placed into the rectum and the prostate is localized using sound waves. Then through the probe, the prostate is anesthetized with local anesthesia so that the biopsy can be performed with minimal pain. Local anesthesia prior to biopsy has become the standard of care and has eliminated the painful experience. The biopsy needle is then passed through the probe and 10-12 passages of the biopsy needle are done. The needle works with a spring-like action to bevel into the prostate gland and remove cores of prostate tissue. These cores are then examined by a pathologist to determine if there is cancer.

Unfortunately there is no absolute certainty that a negative biopsy rules out prostate cancer. Approximately 20% of cancers can be missed on the initial biopsy. Therefore, all patients need to know that even if the initial biopsy is negative they should continue to see their urologist every six months for a repeat rectal and a repeat PSA exams. A second biopsy will be advised over time if the PSA level continues to rise or if the prostate feels different from the original rectal exam. Two or even three biopsy sessions can sometimes be performed on the same patient before a prostate cancer is detected.

In screening for prostate cancer we want PSA values to be in the normal range. Studies show, however, that even with PSA values elevated between 4 ng/ml to 10 ng/ml, 70% of these men still will not have prostate cancer. With PSA values between 10 ng/ml -20 ng/ml, 50% of these men will still not have prostate cancer. Obviously, these statistics demonstrate that the PSA value can be elevated in a great number of men who do not have cancer.

Because of this high percentage of "false elevations," especially in men with either symptomatic or asymptomatic prostatitis, I place my patients on the Krisiloff Diet for 4-6 weeks before I recommend biopsy. Subsequently, a repeat PSA is performed. I assure the patient that waiting 4-6 weeks will not cause harm even if cancer exits. Prostate cancer changes over years and a delay of 4-6 weeks to make the diagnosis will not have negative impacts. Hundreds of my patients who originally presented with an elevated PSA had their PSA value return to the normal range with the Krisiloff Diet, and therefore did not need a biopsy.

When a patient has an elevated PSA, and the PSA returns to normal with the diet, the patient must also understand the need to stay on the Krisiloff Diet and to return to see me every six months. At these return intervals, the patient will have a repeat PSA and a repeat rectal exam. Only if the PSA goes back into the abnormal range, or if on rectal exams, there is a change, will these patients undergo a biopsy.

Since a negative first biopsy of the prostate can miss prostate cancer 20% of the time, these patients must also be followed carefully. In patients with a negative first biopsy, the original elevated PSA level serves as the baseline. These patients are followed every six months with repeat rectal exams, and repeat PSA tests. If there is a change in the feel of the prostate, or if the PSA's values rise significantly from the original PSA "baseline" level, then a repeat prostate biopsy is indicated.

At this juncture, the Krisiloff Diet can also play an important role in preventing unnecessary second biopsies. After a negative first biopsy, I always tell the patient to stay on my diet and see me for periodic careful follow-up. For many of my patients, the PSA remains stable and does not continue to rise from a progressive inflammatory condition. Therefore, the diet helps these patients avoid an unnecessary repeat biopsy

Prostate Specific Antigen (PSA) Case Experiences

Peter is a 43 year old veterinarian. In January 2007, he was referred for a PSA of 4.0 ng/ml. He had no voiding symptoms but had a boggy prostate on rectal exam compatible with prostate inflammation. Therefore, rather than an immediate biopsy, he was started on the Krisiloff Diet.

He returned one month later and now his prostate was of a normal consistency and was 50% smaller to palpation. His PSA on repeat was 1.6 ng/m. He is now followed every six onths and the prostate has remained normal on rectal exam. Repeat PSA testing has been 1.6 ng/ml in July 2007 and 1.4 ng/ml in December 2007. He remains totally committed to the Krisiloff Diet.

John is a 63 year old mechanic. When he first was referred in 1997, he had a PSA of 7 ng/ml, and his prostate felt firm on rectal exam. Because of his concern and anxiety, he wanted to proceed directly with a biopsy.

A biopsy was performed and the pathology showed only inflammation. There was no evidence of cancer. With the biopsy as assurance, he now agreed to go on the Krisiloff Diet, and he is seen every six months for a rectal exam and repeat PSA.

Over the last 10 years, he has stayed on the Krisiloff Diet, and the PSA has remained in the 3.7 ng/ml (at its highest) to 2.1 ng/ml (at its lowest). The most recent PSA measurements have been 2.2 ng/ml, 2.1 ng/ml, 2.4 ng/ml, and 2.6 ng/ml. After the original biopsy and while on the diet, the original prostate firmness disappeared, and for the last 10 years, the prostate has remained smooth, soft and benign in its feel.

Carl is a 58 year old airplane mechanic who came to me in 1992 for problems with daytime urine frequency. He was urinating every one to two hours. Carl also had burning with urination and was getting up from his sleep four to five times a night to go to the bathroom..

On the rectal exam, I felt a normal prostate. His PSA test was 3.2. Carl started the Krisiloff Diet, and one month later all his symptoms were gone. He would then return to me once a year for a rectal exam and a PSA test. Every man over the age of 50 should be followed this way since prostate cancer has become the number one cancer in men. The recommendation is to have a rectal exam and PSA test every year.

In October 1995, Carl's PSA suddenly went up to 4.4. He told me that he was not on the Krisiloff Diet at this time. My rectal exam of the prostate felt normal so rather than rush to do a biopsy of the prostate, I simply suggested strict compliance with the Krisiloff Diet and a repeat PSA in one month. Carl went back on the diet, and one month later his PSA was 3.3. He was now a believer in the Krisiloff Diet. He has stayed strictly on the diet, and his most recent PSA in October 1997 was 3.2. He has no urinary symptoms and his rectal exam shows a completely normal prostate.

George is a 60 year old physician who has a strong family history of prostate cancer. His father died of prostate cancer at the age of 55. His family history and the fear of prostate cancer has brought him to me for a yearly PSA test. His PSA results have always been in the 1.9 range.

Then suddenly, his PSA jumped to 4.2. George was also noticing some discomfort in the groin area, and he was experiencing some discomfort with urination.

Because his prostate felt normal on the rectal exam, I recommended to George that he not rush into a biopsy. Instead, I suggested the Krisiloff Diet and that the PSA test would be repeated in one month. If the PSA was still elevated, we would then do a biopsy. He was not a believer at first, but he went along with my suggestion since his prostate felt normal on the rectal exam.

One month after starting the Krisiloff Diet, he returned and the PSA was now down to 2.9. Because of his family history, he was still concerned that perhaps this last test was not accurate so he stayed on the diet and had another repeat PSA one month later. This PSA result was 2.1.

I am happy to add that all his discomforts have disappeared.

13: PSA AND THE KRISILOFF DIET TO TREAT RECURRENT PROSTATE CANCER

The PSA test is not specific when screening patients for prostate cancer, but its accuracy to detect prostate cancer recurrence in patients previously treated for prostate cancer approaches 100%. And this is another area where the Krisiloff Diet can play a major role.

In appropriate patients, prostate cancer is usually treated with either a radical prostatectomy or with radiation therapy. Radical prostatectomy is the surgical removal of the prostate gland, while radiation therapy is performed in one of two ways. The first method for radiation is with traditional external therapy. The second method is called brachytherapy. With this technique, needles are placed into the prostate under anesthesia. Radioactive pellets (called "seeds") are placed into the prostate through the needles where they remain permanently. The pellets deliver radiation, usually over a period of 56 days, and then become inert. Both methods of radiation achieve the same long-term results, but in the external method, the patient must have treatments once daily, five days a week, over a period of about eight weeks. In brachytherapy the treatment is delivered in one day, but the side effects are greater for the first few months then when compared to those with external therapy.

Studies show that giving hormone therapy in select patients prior to radiation improves the cure rate with radiation by as much as 25% over radiation alone. So today, hormone therapy for several months followed with radiation has become the standard of care for these groups. There are no proven benefits for hormones prior to surgery; therefore, hormone therapy is not given to patients who choose surgery.

When radical prostatectomy is successful, the PSA comes down to 0.1 ng/ml and stay there permanently. With successful radiation therapy, the PSA should get down to 1.0 ng/ml or less. Studies also show that if after radiation, the PSA comes to 0.5 ng/ml or less, there is a higher probability of long-term cure. The PSA is usually measured every six months when following patients with previous prostate cancer therapy.

When PSA measurements stay in these desired ranges, there is little chance of prostate cancer recurrence. But if the values start to climb above these levels, this indicates that the prostate cancer has returned. The time interval it takes for the PSA level to double in value is also critical. We call this PSA doubling time. For patients where the PSA value changes rapidly, serious problems often occur. If the numerical measure of the PSA doubles in six to nine months or less, it is likely this patient will eventually have clinical manifestations of prostate cancer recurrence or death. However, if the rate change is slower, this might suggest better long term survival. For better accuracy, the numerical doubling time is based on three separate PSA values, done every three months.

When the PSA starts to rise after previous curative treatment, important decisions need to be made. There are select cases when radiation therapy can be given to patients who formerly had radical prostatectomies but success is about 40% in curing the recurrence. For patients with past radiation therapy, more radiation cannot be given and surgery to remove a prior radiated prostate is possible but extremely difficult, and has a low rate of cure. There is a treatment called cryosurgery which some recommend in this situation.

With increasing PSA after prior curative therapy, hormone therapy becomes the treatment of choice, but the timing of when to start is controversial. The rationale for hormone therapy is that prostate cancer cells need male hormones (testosterone) for growth. By removing testosterone, the cancer's progression is slowed but not eradicated. There are two methods used to block testosterone. The more common method is with the use of injections. This approach stops the secretion of testosterone from the testicles by blocking pathways for the body to produce testosterone. The other method for eliminating testosterone is to surgically remove the testicles; the organ where the testosterone is produced. This requires an outpatient surgery. Injections require periodic visits for repeat shots for the rest of the patient's life. With testicular removal, there is no further need for periodic hormone treatments and the overall cost for treatment is much less. Eventually, however, hormone therapy loses its effectiveness as the cancer cells become independent from hormone control. At this point chemotherapy becomes appropriate.

Once the PSA starts to rise after previous definitive treatment with either surgery or radiation, the critical decision becomes whether or not these patients need immediate initiation of hormone therapy (advocates call this "early treatment") or whether the same results can be achieved with holding off hormone therapy until the patient actually shows symptoms of cancer progression (advocates call this "late treatment). No study has ever shown that beginning hormone therapy "early" when the PSA first begins to rise has benefit in prolonging survival, versus holding hormone therapy until "later", when symptoms manifest themselves with either weight loss or bone pain.

Hormone therapy is not without major risks. Recently, heart problems and diabetes have been recognized as possible side effects in some people on hormone therapy for prolonged periods. It has also been known for many years that hormones can be associated with bone loss, osteoporosis and increase risks for hip fracture. Sexual dysfunction, muscular changes and mental cognitive changes are also associated with hormone use.

I personally do not advocate "early" hormone treatment for recurrent prostate cancer, but rather believe that delaying treatment until "later" in carefully selected patients can be just as effective. Here again, the Krisiloff Diet helps play a role in my decision on when to start hormones. Studies suggest that cancer does not progress as well in an anti-inflammatory environment, and from clinical experience, my diet is basically a natural anti-inflammatory diet. I would not advocate avoiding traditional treatments, but adding the Krisiloff Diet in the early cancer-recurrent environment can be helpful.

When the PSA first starts to rise, I talk to my patients about the importance of the Krisiloff Diet for its anti-inflammatory effect. The patients are then followed carefully every 3 months. They are followed with attention to their symptoms and the rate of change in their PSA. I have many patients in my practice who have had a slowing of the PSA rate from a rapid progression to a slower progression while strictly maintaining the Krisiloff Diet. These patients can then be followed carefully without the need to rush to hormonal therapy. If these patients maintain a slow increase in PSA changes they can safely be followed without any intervention. This certainly delays the serious side effects associated with hormone therapy. However, if these patients demonstrate a significant change in the velocity of the PSA doubling time or if these patients are not getting along well, then hormonal therapy can be started at that point.

The Krisiloff Diet has been helpful for many of my patients. In essence, the diet seems to work as a natural anti-inflammatory method to slow the progression of their cancer.

Krisiloff Diet and Recurrent Prostate Cancer – Case Experiences

L.S. was 67 years old in May 1987 when he had a radical prostatectomy for a Gleason 7 prostate cancer. The final pathology demonstrated that the cancer invaded the adjacent seminal vesicles, often a poor prognosis. In May 1987, he received post-operative radiation therapy for his more extensive disease, but the effectiveness of radiation in this situation is still debated.

In April 1989, his PSA was 0.8 ng/ml, suggesting that cancer cells were still active and present. At this point the Krisiloff Diet, but no other therapy was started.

From May 1990 until May 1993, the PSA measurements stayed around 0.8 ng/ml. In 1994, his PSA was 1.5 ng/ml, but from then until May 2006, on the Krisiloff Diet only, his PSA stayed in the range between 1.5 ng/ml and 2.3 ng/ml. In October 2006, it was 4.0 ng/ml and in October 2007, it was 7.3 ng/ml.

For the last 20 years and now at age 87, on the Krisiloff Diet only, the patient remains active, healthy and has never experienced clinical signs of prostate cancer recurrence. He knows that hormone therapy might be necessary in the future, but only if clinical problems develop.

H.W. underwent a radical prostatectomy and post-operative radiation for a Gleason 6 prostate cancer with seminal vesicle involvement in July 1986 at age 70 after a hard prostate had been found on rectal exam. His PSA stayed at 0.2 ng/ml until June 1992 when it was 0.4 ng/ml. At this point he was started on the Krisiloff Diet. In July 1996, his PSA was 1.3 ng/ml and stayed between 1.3 ng/ml and 2.5 ng/ml until April 2005. In November 2005, it was 3.1 ng/ml and between then and April 2008, it has risen only to 4.2 ng/ml.

The patient is now 92 years old and has never received any therapy except for the Krisiloff Diet. He remains active and has never demonstrated any clinical problems of prostate cancer.

14: DO ALL PROSTATE CANCERS NEED TO BE TREATED, AND WHEN CAN THE KRISILOFF DIET HELP?

Many urologists believe that prostate cancers in appropriately selected men do not need treatment if the patient's life expectancy is less than 10 years. Especially if their prostate cancer is not aggressive and if their PSA is not changing at a rapid rate. One study has shown that in many men with prostate cancer, there can be a 14 year interval from their initial PSA elevation until their death from the prostate cancer. The American Urology Association has suggestions that even say in men over the age of 75, routine screening for PSA is not necessary or beneficial.

By age 80, approximately 50% of men have evidence of prostate cancer on autopsy studies, yet only 6% of these men die because of their prostate cancer. This demonstrates that many men live with their prostate cancer and die from something else such as heart disease, diabetes, stroke, or other types of cancer. In properly selected men, aggressive treatment of prostate cancer can prove to be disabling, costly, and of no benefit.

From this knowledge, urologists have begun to question whether each and every prostate cancer patient needs to be treated. "Are there insignificant prostate cancers?" Even in younger patients, they are beginning to ask, "Are we doing more good or more harm, by treating prostate cancers that are not highly aggressive?"

When a prostate biopsy is done, the tissue from the biopsy specimen is examined by the pathologist. The pathologist not only determines that prostate cancer is present, but they also evaluate the nucleus of the cancer cells to designate how aggressive that specific cancer will be. From their evaluation, they can assign what is called a Gleason score. The appearance of the cancer cell allows them to assign a specific standardized Gleason score.

The Gleason score can then act as a surrogate to try and identify how aggressive that individual's cancer can be. A prostate cancer assigned a Gleason score of 6 is considered a low risk cancer, meaning it is less aggressive and therefore less likely to have short term harm. A tumor with a Gleason score of 7 is considered a moderate risk cancer. A Gleason score of 8 or 9 is considered a high risk cancer and increases the risk for that individual patient eventually dying from his prostate cancer.

In addition to examining the biopsy specimens for a Gleason score, the pathologist also reviews the entire biopsy tissue submitted to determine the actual amount of cancer found on the total specimen. If only a small percent of the biopsy specimen shows cancer, this could be useful as a surrogate to suggest there is actually a small amount of prostate cancer in the patient's entire prostate. Likewise if a large percent of cancer is found on the biopsy specimen, this could suggest a much larger amount of cancer is present in the patient's prostate, and therefore, this patient might need more aggressive treatment.

Prostate cancer treatment with either surgery or radiation is not without significant risk. Impotency and urine incontinence are major problems associated with both of these treatments. If aggressive unnecessary treatment could be avoided, lifetime debilitating problems could be avoided as well. With this in mind, the concept of "active surveillance" is being discussed more frequently.

The concept of "active surveillance" is emerging as perhaps a better way to determine which patients truly need aggressive treatments, and which patients can be followed conservatively. A recent study followed appropriately selected patients with active surveillance for their prostate cancer and demonstrated that only 36% of the patients required therapy after almost six and a half years of follow-up.

Active surveillance could be considered for patients with a low risk Gleason score and low volume of cancer on their initial biopsy. These patients do not require that a decision on cancer treatment be made immediately. Instead, they can be followed very carefully. These patients must understand however that they remain at risk, and that close and prolonged surveillance is required. Most prostate cancers do not change rapidly. Therefore, a program with properly selected patients who choose to delay treatment for a matter of a few months or even years will not necessarily change their probability of cure, and in many cases, these patients might be those who never need treatment.

In my practice, carefully selected patients are informed about all options for treatment including surgery, radiation or active surveillance. If they choose active surveillance, they must understand that repeat biopsies and PSA tests are required periodically. Careful follow-up is a must to ensure that larger amounts of prostate cancer or higher risk cancers are subsequently not found.

The first repeat biopsy is done at three months, and if the clinical situation allows, repeat biopsies are done six months later, and then once each year. The patient is also seen every six months for PSA blood tests. If there is a significant change in the blood test, then a repeat biopsy is necessary at that time.

It is thought that prostate cancer does not progress as rapidly in an anti-inflammatory environment. Therefore, in my practice, all patients under active surveillance are on the Krisiloff Diet because of its anti-inflammatory properties.

I caution anyone who is considering active surveillance to discuss this approach carefully with their urologist. They must be certain that their doctor will agree to the proper program for many years of follow-up. They must also understand their own responsibility for appropriate follow-up.

Do All Prostate Cancers Need Treatment – Case Experiences

Scott is a 50 years old who works at a book store. In May 2003, he had a biopsy for a PSA of 5.3 ng/ml. The pathologist reported a prostate cancer with a Gleason score of 6 and only 2% of the biopsy specimen showed cancer. Because of the low grade risk with a Gleason score of 6 and a small volume of cancer, all options were discussed with the patient. Although, surgery and radiation were strong options in a young man, he chose active surveillance and was placed on the Krisiloff Diet.

As part of the careful follow-up, he had repeat biopsies in August 2003, March 2004, September 2004, September 2005, March 2007, and March 2008. All biopsies were negative. In addition, the PSA has fluctuated from the original 5.3 ng/ml in 2003 to 8.5 ng/ml in 2002, and most recently back to 6.7 ng/ml in March 2008.

He continues to be followed carefully and understands that more aggressive treatments might be necessary if the clinical situation should change.

In April 1995, **Jack** was a 64 year old businessman. At that time, a PSA of 5.2 ng/ml led to a biopsy. The biopsy showed a Gleason 6 prostate cancer with only 5% of the biopsy specimen showing cancer. Because of a low risk in this situation, and after all options were discussed, the patient chose active surveillance. He was also placed on the Krisiloff Diet.

Repeat biopsies in June 1995 and February 1996, were negative. A fourth biopsy in March 1997, showed a Gleason 6 with less than 1% of the biopsy tissue showing cancer. But at this point with the patient on the Krisiloff Diet, the PSA was now 1.0 ng/ml. A repeat biopsy in October 1999, was negative with a PSA of 1.5 ng/ml.

A repeat biopsy in February 2001, was also negative. After this biopsy, the patient developed a post-biopsy infection and therefore did not want to undergo further biopsies. However, he continues to be followed carefully. His most recent PSA in March 2008, was 3.0 ng/ml, and on rectal exam the prostate continues to feel normal.

The patient is now 76 years old and continues to be seen every six months for rectal exams and PSA tests.

James is a retired gentleman. In 2002, at the age of 76, he was referred to me with a PSA of 33 ng/ml. I strongly advised for a prostate biopsy, but he did not want one at that time.

In January 2004, he developed urine retention --- a situation where he was unable to urinate. The rectal exam did not suggest prostate cancer, but after surgery to relieve the problem, the pathology report showed a Gleason 6 cancer of the prostate with 13% of the specimen showing cancer. His PSA at this time was 41 ng/ml. After surgery, he voided normally and had no other symptoms. At this time, he was strongly advised to go on the Krisiloff Diet, but he was not compliant.

By September 2006, still with no symptoms, his PSA climbed to 50 ng/ml. At this time, he agreed to become 100% compliant with the Krisiloff Diet. Hormone therapy was discussed, but it was decided to hold off hormones until the clinical situation would definitely indicate a need, such as bone pain or loss of weight.

In November 2006, his PSA was 58 ng/ml. His most recent PSA in February 2008 was 58 ng/ml. He stays on the Krisiloff Diet, still has no symptoms, and is living a normal life. He is followed carefully, and knows that if problems develop, he will need hormone therapy.

15: THE KRISILOFF DIET AND THE PREVENTION OF PROSTATE CANCER

Prostate cancer is the second-leading cause of cancer death in men. Approximately 230,000 men are newly diagnosed yearly with prostate cancer, and each year there are approximately 29,000 men who die from it. During their lifetime, one of every six men will develop prostate cancer. With such a significant toll in lives, misery and cost, think how enormous the achievement would be if there was a way to prevent or decrease this "plague."

Presently, there is great interest in the association between inflammation, and its connection to cancer. Major changes are also occurring in how the medical world looks upon prostate inflammation and its potential to cause prostate cancer. In the last three years, there have been three major articles in the urology journals suggesting a possible link between inflammation and prostate cancer.

In the past when I spoke with my patients about prostatitis, I always told them it would affect the quality of their everyday life, but there was no evidence to suggest it could cause significant health problems. Now, because of the recent articles, I educate them about the possible link between chronic prostatitis and prostate cancer. We also talk about how the Krisiloff Diet could be a way to prevent prostate cancer because of its demonstrated anti-inflammatory properties and its ability to cure chronic prostatitis,

The body responds to acute inflammation, by releasing compounds called oxygen free radicals. These compounds fight inflammation and help the body protect itself. However, in situations with chronic inflammation, oxygen free radicals are no longer helpful, but instead attack DNA in cells leading to cell mutation. Recent studies have shown that in chronic prostatitis, oxygen free radicals are toxic to cells and could possibly be implicated in prostate cancer development.

Often when biopsies are done for detecting prostate cancer, rather than showing cancer they show other different pathological conditions. One of these pathological findings is called proliferative inflammatory atrophy (PIA). PIA is found in areas of the prostate associated with chronic inflammation. PIA develops when cells attempt to regenerate prostate tissue damaged by chronic inflammation.

Proliferative inflammatory atrophy can also be found in biopsy specimens in close association with another pathological process called high grade PIN (prostate intraepithelial neoplasm). It is believed by many that high grade PIN is a precursor to prostate cancer.

Possible Pathway for Prostatitis to Prostate Cancer

Chronic Prostate Inflammation
↓
Proliferative Inflammatory Antrophy (PIA)
↓
Prostate Intraepithelial neoplasm (PIN)
↓
Prostate Cancer

While there is no definite proof that inflammation leads to prostate cancer, there are growing suggestions about this connection. In prostate cancer there are elevated levels of substances called prostaglandins. Recent studies have implicated prostaglandins in the development and progression of cancers because they can cause uncontrolled cell proliferation. To produce prostaglandin, a chemical precursor called cyclooxygenase is required. Cyclooxygenase exists in two forms: Cox-1 and Cox-2. Cox-2 is found in cancers, including prostate cancer at higher levels than in normal tissue. Many believe that suppression of Cox-2 can lead to suppression of cancer growth through an anti-inflammatory effect.

Possible Pathway for Inflammation Causing Cancer

Cyclooxygenase (Cox-1 and Cox-2)
↓
Prostaglandins
↓
Uncontrolled Cellular Proliferation
↓
Cancer

A class of drugs called non-steroidal anti-inflammatory drugs (NSAID) function as Cox-2 inhibitors. The most famous of the Cox-2 inhibitors is Vioxx ---commonly used by patients with arthritis for its anti-inflammatory effects. Vioxx was recently removed from the market because of its potential serious effects on the cardiovascular system. Until its removal, there were ongoing trials to use Vioxx for prostate cancer control, because of its known anti inflammatory properties. The theory being that inflammation produces increased cyclooxygenase and prostaglandins and that these compounds promote cancer and cancer growth. The Cox-2 inhibitors would, therefore, inhibit this, and hopefully slow the growth of cancer.

The most significant study linking prostate inflammation and prostate cancer may be from Case-Western Reserve University Hospital, published in the September 2006 Journal of Urology. This study was the first to suggest an increased relationship of prostatitis and prostate cancer in the same individuals. Doctors biopsied men with elevated PSA levels to screen for prostate cancer. From the biopsy results, they were able to split these men into two distinct groups. Men in group 1 had elevated PSAs and their biopsies showed chronic inflammation but no evidence of cancer. Men in group 2 had no evidence of inflammation, no evidence of cancer, and no definite explanation for their elevated PSAs.

Within five years they then re-biopsied these same men. In the men with chronic inflammation on their original biopsy (Group 1), 20% of these men now showed prostate cancer. In the group without inflammation (Group 2), only 6% of men were found to have cancer on the re-biopsy. The conclusion of this study: "chronic inflammation may be a significant risk factor for cancer of the prostate."

For close to 30 years, and in thousands of men, I have cured prostatitis using the Krisiloff Diet. The Krisiloff Diet has continually shown that it can prevent and eliminate prostatitis. Therefore, it seems logical that if the Krisiloff Diet can prevent chronic inflammation, it might also prevent changes in the prostate resulting from inflammation that could lead to prostate cancer.

I have strong clinical experience that I can prevent prostatitis and cure prostatitis through diet alone. Therefore, I am willing to say that the Krisiloff Diet should be used as a way to potentially prevent or control prostate cancer. Just as 40 years ago people spoke about stopping cigarette smoking to prevent lung cancer, the anti-inflammatory effects of the Krisiloff Diet will hopefully help to decrease and prevent the occurrence of prostate cancer in the future.

16: GASTROESOPHAGEAL REFLUX DISEASE (GERD) AND THE KRISILOFF DIET

Gastroesophageal reflux disease (GERD) causes stomach problems for millions of people. Commonly known as "heartburn," approximately 15 million Americans have symptoms every day and some 60 million Americans have symptoms at least once monthly.

As part of normal anatomy, there are muscles called sphincter muscles located in many different systems throughout our bodies. One such sphincter muscle is located between the esophagus and the stomach. Its purpose is to prevent stomach content from refluxing or going back up into the esophagus.

With GERD, this specific sphincter becomes weakened and defective. Because this muscle is not functioning properly, it allows stomach content to flow back into the esophagus. Gastroesophageal Reflux Disease is simply stomach acid regurgitating into the esophagus causing a painful burning effect on the esophagus. Heartburn, or "acid indigestion," is the result of GERD. Sleep apnea, chronic cough and adult-onset asthma can also be associated with this problem.

When GERD becomes chronic, cells lining the esophagus undergo inflammatory changes caused by the acid. These chronic inflammatory changes can then develop into a condition called "Barrett's esophagus.". Barrett's esophagus is a pre-malignant condition found in about 10% of people suffering from GERD for five years or longer. 5-10% of people with Barrett's esophagus will also go on to develop esophageal cancer.

Approximately 14,000 people develop esophageal cancer each year. In its early stages, esophageal cancer has no symptoms, so it is difficult to diagnose. Therefore, successful treatment is limited. As the cancer grows it narrows the esophagus, making swallowing difficult or painful, but now it is advanced and therefore, difficult to cure. Patient survival at five years is estimated to be only 15%. Studies suggest that esophageal cancer is the fastest-growing cancer in America today.

With minor heartburn problems, patients use over-the-counter medications, such as Mylanta and Rolaids. These medications neutralize the acid that refluxes from the stomach. For more serious problems, medicines are given which actually reduce the acid content produced by the stomach.

While pharmaceutical means are effective in reducing the amount of acid that refluxes, they do not stop the reflux. Reflux still occurs because the sphincter muscle is still defective, and medicines have no effect on strengthening the defective sphincter muscle. Additionally, because medications do not prevent reflux, they might actually make the situation worse ---painful symptoms are eliminated, but with less acid, the stomach contents become alkaline, and some doctors believe alkaline reflux could be worse than acid reflux in damaging the esophagus.

It is known that certain foods and drinks actually weaken the sphincter muscle and therefore, allow reflux. This probably explains why the Krisiloff Diet has been effective for hundreds of my patients suffering from GERD ---through dietary changes only. Medical studies show that caffeine and alcohol weaken the sphincter muscle. Rather than changing acid content and only masking the problem, the Krisiloff Diet removes those foods and drinks and specifically cures the problem by allowing the sphincter muscle to become normal again. With a restored normally functioning sphincter muscle, people will no longer reflux.

The experiences gained from my urological patients allowed me to use the Krisiloff Diet for the prevention of heartburn and reflux. Over the years, hundreds of my patients on the Krisiloff Diet for urinary problems came back and told me that they also no longer suffered from their stomach and heartburn problems. In the same way that I gained knowledge in curing urinary problems ---by simply listening to my patients, I came to understand what could work for their stomach problems as well.

Gastroesophageal Reflux Disease (GERD) - Case Experience

John is a 55 year old real estate agent who first came to see me because of urinary symptoms. He complained of frequent urination, difficulty in starting his stream and urinating two or three times each night. In addition, he had a long history of esophageal reflux and was taking medicine for this problem. Because he was young and had a small prostate on rectal exam, I felt he suffered from prostatitis and started him on the Krisiloff Diet.

On his return visit, one month later, he no longer had any significant voiding problems. In addition, he had stopped the medication at my suggestion, and he related that he no longer felt symptoms of heartburn.

Presently, he is not on medications and remains free of all symptoms for over two years by simply adhering to my suggestions.

Letter from d.M.M.

01-Oct-2004

Dr. Milton Krisiloff
2001 Santa Monica Blvd. Santa Monica, CA. 90404
Dear Dr. Krisiloff
   I am cured. I am also deeply indebted to you in your ability to diagnose my condition and perscribe the "krisiloff diet".
   The condition of blood in my urine (gross hematuria) along with extreme pain, plus waking 5/6 times during the night to urinate is gone.
   You cured three for three - inflamation of the prostate, no more blood in the urine, and my psa count dropped to within a normal count of 3.5.
   In addition, my heart-burn is gone forever along with the loss -
Of about 15 lbs.
I will live by your diet.

Sincerely,
D.M.M.
(Marina Del Rey, California)

17: RHEUMATOID ARTHRITIS AND THE KRISILOFF DIET

Approximately forty-eight million Americans suffer from rheumatoid arthritis, and the cost for its treatments and in lost productivity approaches $64 billion per year. It is considered the leading cause of disability in our country. Over the next decade rheumatoid arthritis is expected to affect 60 million Americans.

Rheumatoid arthritis is caused by inflammation affecting the bones and joints of our bodies. Our joints are covered by a spongy material called cartilage which helps lubricate them allowing for movement without pain. When inflammation occurs, cartilage undergoes change, and loses its protective qualities. This results in the pain, stiffness and difficulty in movement that we associate with rheumatoid arthritis.

For many years aspirin, because of its anti-inflammatory properties, was the treatment of choice for dealing with arthritic inflammation. The problem with aspirin, however, was that in many people it caused stomach irritation and internal bleeding.

In an attempt to overcome these serious side effects, a new class of drugs was developed. These drugs are classified as non-steroidal anti-inflammatory drugs (NSAID). The hope was that they would be a major advancement in treating arthritis without the side effects of aspirin. However, recent studies have suggested that there could be problems with these drugs as well. Vioxx (an NSAID drug) was recently removed from the market due to the possible linkage of Vioxx with serious, and sometimes deadly, side effects associated with heart attacks and strokes.

In addition to the NSAID drugs, other classes of drugs have been developed. These target specific inflammatory agents to treat rheumatoid arthritis. While these drugs have shown dramatic effectiveness in helping people, the major disadvantage is their expense. These new medications require frequent injections at a cost of two thousand dollars per month. Just think of that - $24,000 per year per individual patient.

Like most things in medicine, early diagnosis and treatment provides the best chance for control or cure. The key is to prevent inflammation from damaging tissue before it turns into a chronic problem with disabling changes. This again is where the Krisiloff Diet can play a major role.

Early treatment and prevention has significant relevance for me on a personal level. Years ago I started to develop joint pains in my fingers, a scenario familiar for many people with early arthritis. As a surgeon, you can imagine my fear about the potential future threat to my career.

One night while dining in an Indian restaurant, eating a spicy curry dish, I felt the sudden onset of severe pain in my fingers. Fortunately, I likened the attack to what many of my patients had previously told me about their experience with their prostatitis attacks. Those most susceptible had often noticed an immediate onset of symptoms when they consumed "forbidden foods" on the Krisiloff Diet.

I immediately recognized that there must be an association between the arthritic flair-up, and the food that I was eating. With this knowledge, I placed myself on the Krisiloff Diet and the arthritis symptoms in my fingers went away within weeks. Because I stayed on the Krisiloff Diet, they have never returned.

Since then, I have seen many patients with urinary symptoms who also have arthritis. If their arthritic problem is early in its development, before chronic tissue changes occur, I always tell them that with the Krisiloff Diet their urinary symptoms will definitely disappear and their arthritis symptoms will likely disappear as well.

Letter from R.S.

Dear Dr. Krisiloff,

As you might recall, prior to seeing you for what turned out to be a case of prostatitis, I was suffering with severe leg pain for over five years. I had seen many doctors and specialists in Los Angeles and had even gone to the Mayo Clinic in Rochester, Minnesota for a full 5 day medical work up. No one could diagnose the source of my leg pain. I cannot even remember the amount of prescription medication I was taking.

After following your diet for several months, not only did the prostatitis clear up but also, to my surprise, the leg pain dissipated and is now completely gone and I am not on any medications. The few times I have broken the diet, especially drinking a cup of coffee, the leg pain comes back within an hour.

R.S. (Glendale, California, 2006)

Letter from J.F.

Dear Dr. Krisiloff,

This is to let you know that I am feeling much better from following your advice to discontinue taking coffee, tea, and chocolate. I was taking Celebrex for my arthritis, Prilosec for my acidity, Lipitor for my high cholesterol, and Hytrin for my enlarged prostate gland, plus an occasional pain remedy.

When I went to see you, I more or less expected you to recommend some expensive treatment or surgery, so I was delighted to hear you recommend less, rather than more, medications. I have followed your advice, and I am happy to say that I am off all of the above medications without any untoward effects. I recommend your advice to all of my friends.

Sincerely,
J.F. (Los Angeles, California, 2004)

Letter to Dr. Krisiloff

The Krisiloff Diet is the only New Year's resolution I have actually kept! The results have been remarkable. Not only did my urinary problems disappear, but so did the GERD I had been experiencing. It seems to me that if the gastroenterologist who told me to limit my coffee to 1-2 cups daily advised his patients to follow the Krisiloff Diet, his practice would be vastly reduced. He suggested a test for Bar-

rett's esophagitis (happily, the HMO didn't approve it) but he should have been recommending the Krisiloff Diet. My discomfort would have been immediately reduced and I wouldn't have had to take Protonix and Prilosec.

But the real surprise of the Krisiloff Diet came when I realized that I was no longer having to take two Advil and half a Vicodin before bedtime in order to stave off awakening at 3 a.m. with "screaming knees." I had tried Celebrex for my knees but it was not helpful, so I had been taking Advil for years, essentially around the clock. The Krisiloff Diet got rid of what I thought was arthritis, an unexpected and significant improvement in my daily life, and I am very appreciative.

Thanks!

18: OTHER MEDICAL CONDITIONS HELPED BY THE KRISILOFF DIET

For 30 years, the Krisiloff Diet has cured urological problems for thousands of my patients. Simultaneously, hundreds of these same patients have been cured of secondary problems such as GERD and arthritis. From these large numbers, I have identified the association between their diseases and their cures in using my diet. For diseases associated with inflammation, the Krisiloff Diet has dramatically demonstrated its effect as an anti-inflammatory diet.

With fewer patients to be as definitive, I have seen miraculous cures for other medical problems as well. Since the Krisiloff Diet is a holistic approach with no harmful effects, it seems logical to consider it for first-line treatment in other diseases where I have seen excellent results. Cures occur rapidly, and it could avoid more invasive and expensive approaches.

While on the Krisiloff Diet, some of my patients with elevated blood pressure have been able to reduce or even eliminate their blood pressure medications. The Krisiloff Diet is not intended for weight loss, but many patients lose 7-10 pounds within weeks of going on the diet. This weight loss may contribute to lowering their blood pressure. We also know that alcohol and caffeine can elevate blood pressure.

Chronic sinusitis, a common problem, has been cured with my diet. Patients have related how they have suffered for years, even on medication, yet nothing helped to cure their sinusitis until they went on the Krisiloff Diet.

Patients with heart palpitations or rapid heartbeats have been cured. Cardiology colleagues tell me that eliminating alcohol and caffeine are often recommended as the first step in treating irregular heart rhythms.

Skin rashes have disappeared with the Krisiloff Diet. Rosacea, a common skin rash, is known to have a link to caffeine. Additionally, patients with Psoriasis have reported improvement to their skin condition with the Krisiloff Diet

People with chronic headaches (even migraines) see tremendous relief with the Krisiloff Diet. Since 10% of Americans suffer from migraines, the effect can be significant. Neurology colleagues inform me there is scientific basis to eliminate caffeine and alcohol for people suffering migraines. Patients often feel they need caffeine to help control headaches, but instead they need to understand that a vicious cycle exists. Caffeine actually contributes to, rather than controls the recurrence of headache cycles. I do warn patients when they initially go on the diet that they might experience symptoms of caffeine withdrawal, and that headaches can occur. But the only way to achieve long term relief from recurrent headaches is to abruptly break from this pattern. After 1-2 weeks the headache symptoms will disappear. The patients will feel better, and the headaches will not return as long as they stay on the diet.

Patients with Multiple Sclerosis have reported to me their improvement in clinical conditions while following my diet.

Finally, I have several patients with the "restless leg" syndrome. They suffer from spasms or twitches in their legs while they sleep. The involuntary movement creates anxiety and significant disruption in their sleep pattern. Within six to eight weeks of going on the Krisiloff Diet, the "restless leg" syndrome has completely disappeared.

Other Medical Conditions Helped by The Krisiloff Diet – Case Experiences

Anna is a 55 year old woman who came to see me because of increased frequency and nocturia three to four times each night. In addition she suffered from migraines, heart palpitations and "esophageal spasms."

She was placed on the Krisiloff Diet because of her urine symptoms. She returned one month later and had no further medical problems. She was then seen six months later, and in addition to no urinary problems, she also was free of migraines, heart palpitations and GERD.

As you can imagine, she was eternally grateful.

Peter is a 45 year old man who came to see me in June 2006 for an elevated PSA of 6.2 ng/ml. He also informed me that he suffered from

GERD and chronic sinusitis. His prostate on exam was benign.

He was started on the Krisiloff Diet and returned in July 2006. His prostate was 50% smaller on rectal exam and still felt benign. His PSA was now 4.2 ng/ml. Because of the change, I suggested he stay on the diet and see me in eight more weeks.

On his return, his PSA was now 3.2 ng/ml, and he was excited to tell me that his GERD and sinusitis were gone. He returned six months later on the diet, and his PSA was now 2.5 ng/ml.

19: CONCLUSION

After reading this book, some will say I have no scientific basis for my claims. I will not dispute this. Yet after thousands of successes and 30 years of experience, I know that it does work and there is no doubt of its effectiveness.

When I initially talk to patients about the Krisiloff Diet, I probably sound like the old "snake oil" salesman because I make so many claims. Their reaction seems to be in either of two schools: skepticism --- they don't believe something so simple can work, or anger --- they resent having to give up food and drinks they feel are so important to their enjoyment. When they leave my office for the first time, I assure them that I have "10,000 patients who believe in the Krisiloff Diet, but it is difficult to find three doctors who do." When most return for subsequent visits, all doubts have vanished.

The diet fulfills one of the most important dictums in all medicine: "Doctor do no harm." In an age when many people want a holistic approach to health care, the Krisiloff Diet is the most holistic treatment ever devised. No cost, no herbs, and no medication ---just the simple elimination of specific items from our diet that I have consistently demonstrated to cause so many different medical problems.

I leave it for the scientists to explain how the Krisiloff Diet works, but it works. Through observation and vast clinical experience, I empirically have discovered the "Holy Grail" for explaining how inflammation can develop in our bodies and cause disease.

The clinical benefits are huge. If inflammation leads to prostate cancer, the diet could be a way to prevent cancer. If inflammation allows prostate cancer to grow more rapidly we might slow its progression or delay treatment in situations where the treatment does not change the chance for survival. If inflammation is responsible for destabilizing cholesterol plaques, leading to heart attacks as some believe, then we have a path to decrease heart disease. If inflammation has a role in Alzheimer's disease or diabetes, as some people think, then a healthy anti-inflammatory diet may be the answer to avoid these debilitating problems.

The Krisiloff Diet has demonstrated great success for 30 years. It is simple, inexpensive, works quickly and poses no risks. It is my hope that people who read this book will consider it as a path to a long and healthy life.

Letter from L.L.

This spring I started on the Krisiloff Diet, not expecting any results, to get rid of my prostate problems which I have had for the last 40 years. To say the least, I am now more than happy to be cured! After all these years of pain and "tons" of medicine, I am now praising every day. And all I did was to leave some habits behind me, and that was hardly any sacrifice.

Thanks for your advice.
L.L. (Portugal, 2006)

APPENDIX

Milligrams of Caffeine in Various Drinks and Chocolate[1]

Coffee:
Espresso, 2 ounces 120
Regular, brewed, 6 ounces 103
Instant, 6 ounces 57
Instant, decaf, 6 ounces 2

Tea:
Black, 6 ounces* 53
Oolong, 6 ounces* 36
Green, 6 ounces* 32
Iced tea, instant, 12 ounces 46

Soft Drinks, 12 ounces:**
Jolt Cola 72
Nehi Maxxvm Cola 70
Sundrop 63
Kick 58
Mountain Dew 55
Mello Yello, Surge 53
Coca-Cola Classic 47
Royal Crown Cola 43
Mr. Pibb, Dr. Pepper, Sunkist Sparkling Lemonade 41
Sunkist Orange 40
Squirt Ruby Red 39
Pepsi 37
A & W Cream Soda 28
Barq's 23
Slice Cola 11

Water, Caffeine Enhanced, 12 ounces:
Java Water 71
Krank 2O 70
Water Joe 46
Aqua Java 43

Juice Drinks, Caffeine Enhanced, 12 ounces:

Java Juice 90
XTC 70

Chocolate:

Baking chocolate, unsweetened, 1 ounce 58
Hershey Special Dark chocolate bar, 1.45 ounces 31
Milk chocolate candy bars, average, 1.55 ounces 11

*Brewed in bag for 3 minutes.
**Diet sodas have roughly the same caffeine as regular versions.

[1]*Source: Los Angeles Times, Feb. 1998 / Consumer Reports on Health, Sept. 1997*

Common Beverages, Foods and Medications Containing Caffeine

Coffee	Tea	Cocoa
Cola Drinks	Dr. Pepper	Mountain Dew
Chocolate	Anacin	Dristan
Empirin	Excedrin	No-Doz

Alcohol means all beverages containing alcohol, including beer and wine. Extremely hot spicy foods include salsa, hot peppers, hot mustards, horseradish, chili, Tabasco, hot sauce and pepperoni.

Hot Spicy Foods Which Are Prohibited

Salsa	Chili	Tobasco
Curry	Hot Mustards	Hot Sauce
Horseradish	Spicy Thai Food	Hot Peppers
Wasabi	Ginger	Spicy Chinese Food
Pepperoni		

It is not necessary to be on a bland diet. Mild spices such as salt, black pepper, onion, salad dressing, or ketchup are not irritants, and it is acceptable to consume these medium spices. Some people have been told by physicians to avoid tomatoes and citrus juice. However, I have not found this necessary and tell my patients it is okay to consume these products.

Mild Spices Allowable On The Krisiloff Diet

Garlic	Spaghetti Sauce	Onion
Pizza (no pepperoni)	Ketchup	Delicatessen Meat
Mild Mustard	Black Pepper	Salad Dressing

GLOSSARY

A

Acute Cystitis - An infection in the urine which is caused by bacteria and requires antibiotics.

Acute Prostatitis - An infection of the prostate gland, usually accompanied by high fevers.

C

Chronic Prostatitis - A chronic inflammation of the prostate gland which is not a true infection and is usually not helped by antibiotics.

C-Reactive Protein - Protein used as markers in inflammation. Level rises during inflammatory processes.

Cyclooxygenase - Enzyme in body. Blockage of cyclooxygenase provides relief from inflammation.

Cytokines - proteins critical for immune responses

D

Dysuria - Pain with urination and / or a burning sensation associated with the act of urination.

E

Enuresis - A clinical word used to describe bed-wetting. Bed-wetting is considered abnormal if it occurs after the age of 6.

Epididymitis - An inflammation of the gland that is next to the testicle. The epididymis gland is where metabolic changes occur in the sperm which is produced by the testicle.

G

GERD - Gastrointestinal reflux disease ---commonly known as heartburn.

Gross Hematuria - Blood in the urine which is visible to the naked eye.

H

hematospermia - Blood in the semen.

hematuria - Blood in the urine.

hesitancy - Difficulty in starting the urine stream. The individual has to wait several seconds before the urine stream starts to flow.

I

incontinence - The involuntary loss of urine causing the undergarments or clothes to become wet.

inflammation - A localized reaction due to irritation or infection. In many cases, inflammation is not due to a true infection and does not require antibiotics.

M

macrophages - cells from white blood cells remove dead cell material.

microscopic hematuria - Blood in the urine that is not visible to the naked eye. It is seen only by microscopic exam.

N

nocturia - Getting up from sleep to urinate. It is abnormal to get up to urinate more than once during the night.

O

oxygen free radicals – Molecules produced in the body that can cause alterations in tissue which can lead to cancer or chronic inflammatory conditions.

P

premature ejaculation - If a man cannot delay ejaculation long enough to satisfy his sexual partner. The ejaculation usually comes too soon --- in 15 to 30 seconds.

Proliferative Inflammatory Atrophy (PIA) – Cellular changes in the prostate which result from chronic inflammation and may be linked to the development of prostate cancer.

Prostate Intraepithelial Neoplasm (PIN) - Changes in prostate tissue where cells show pre-malignant features but not definite cancer.

Prostate Specific Antigen (PSA) - A blood test to screen for prostate cancer. PSA is a protein produced by the prostate. The PSA test is not specific for prostate cancer. It can be falsely elevated if one has an inflamed or enlarged prostate.

Prostatitis - An inflammation of the prostate gland. The prostate gland makes fluid for ejaculation.

R

Rosacea – A common skin condition which causes redness on the forehead, cheeks and nose.

S

stress incontinence - The involuntary loss of urine during activity such as running, coughing, jumping or sneezing.

U

urethra - The tube that exits the bladder and carries the urine out from the bladder.

urethral syndrome - An inflammation of the urethra in women which leads to significant urinary problems.

urgency incontinence - The sudden need to urinate followed by the inability to hold the urine and the individual wets him or herself.

urine frequency - An abnormal increase in the urinary pattern. An individual who needs to urinate less than every two hours has urine frequency.

urine urgency - The need to urinate comes on suddenly and the person feels like they cannot hold the urine back.